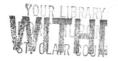

SEP   2006

Lessons
IN MORTALITY

Lessons IN MORTALITY

DOCTORS AND PATIENTS
STRUGGLING TOGETHER

ALLEN B. WEISSE, M.D.

UNIVERSITY OF MISSOURI PRESS   COLUMBIA AND LONDON

Library of Congress Cataloging-in-Publication Data

Weisse, Allen B.
  Lessons in mortality : doctors and patients struggling together
/ Allen B. Weisse.
      p.   cm.
  Summary: "Writing frankly, Weisse discusses how doctors and
patients of cancer, heart disease, stroke, infectious disease, AIDS, and
other dire diagnoses deal with illness in the twenty-first century,
considering, in turn, how such factors as specialization, rising costs,
managed care, the indurance industry, and litigation has changed the
practice of medicine"—Provided by publisher.
  ISBN-13: 978-0-8262-1666-3 (hard cover : alk. paper)
  ISBN-10: 0-8262-1666-8 (hard cover : alk. paper)
   1. Critically ill—Psychology. 2. Critically ill—Conduct of life.
3. Physician and patient. 4. Health behavior.
   [DNLM: 1. Attitude to Death—Personal Narratives. 2. Physician-
Patient Relations—Personal Narratives. 3. Death—Personal
Narratives. 4. Physician's Practice Patterns—Personal Narratives.
5. Sick Role—Personal Narratives. W 62 W432L 2006] I. Title.
  R726.5.W454 2006
  616—dc22

                                                        2006007806

∞™This paper meets the requirements of the
American National Standard for Permanence of Paper
for Printed Library Materials, Z39.48, 1984.

Designer: Jennifer Cropp
Typesetter: Crane Composition, Inc.
Printer and binder: Thomson-Shore, Inc.
Typefaces: Minion, Schneidler, and Shelley

To all my

patients

and to all my

doctors

Contents

1. INTRODUCTION   1

2. LANCE ARMSTRONG AND ME   6

3. THE CROCK   36

4. DEVOTION   43

5. THE IRON MAN   46

6. WASTE   55

7. MARKING TIME AT HILLCREST HOME   58

8. THE CASE OF THE BAFFLING BOY: CHAPTER ONE   64

9. EDDY   72

10. SMART ASS   77

11. VICTIMS ALL   81

12. THE END OF THE ROAD   101

13. MODERN MEDICINE   111

14. THE SURVIVOR   115

15. A MAN WHAT AM   122

16. OTHER FACES OF AIDS   128

17. ON DYING WITH DIGNITY—AND A DIAGNOSIS   140

18. THE GIFT   151

19. TIME (OVERDUE) FOR A CHANGE   159

20. STROKE   166

21. A LETTER   178

Lessons
IN MORTALITY

Oh wad some power the giftie gie us
To see orsels as ithers see us!

—Robert Burns (1759-1796)

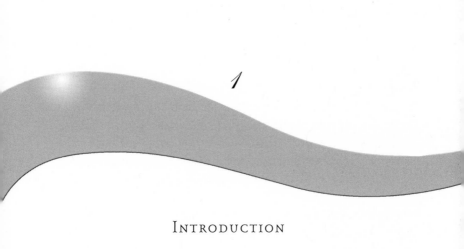

1

INTRODUCTION

Norman Rockwell was an American original. Although the cognoscenti of the art world always looked down their collective noses at his work, the rest of us viewed with affection all those *Saturday Evening Post* covers that provided the widest outlet for his illustrations, spanning a great part of the last century.

Not long ago, wandering through the museum in Stockbridge, Massachusetts, that houses much of his collected work, I wondered if the homespun, apple-pie vision of America that he represented to us ever really existed or if it merely was what he and his audience nostalgically wished it ought to have been. As a physician, I was particularly struck by his depiction of the doctor—a country doctor, of course—aging, with wisps of unruly white hair over a broad pate; ruddy but cherubic in countenance; chubbily bulging out of his rumpled gray vested suit; and listening with mock intensity, his stethoscope pressed to the chest of the rag doll presented to him by the anxious tiny wisp of a girl before him. In another illustration he appears in profile, leaning forward in his chair to reassure two young parents before him that the child they have brought to him will surely be all right.

No less an idealized portrait of the family doctor was produced by the British artist Sir Samuel Luke Fildes in 1891. Here a bearded physician, looking much like the mature Pasteur, keeps a midnight vigil at the bedside of a seriously ill child. The lamplight reflects in the doctor's features the kind of warmth, compassion, and devotion that all patients must seek in their physicians.

Fildes's and Rockwell's contrasting but complementary depictions of "the good doctor" must have been ingrained upon the consciousness of generations of patients. Copies of Fildes's painting, in particular, must have been as familiar to doctors' offices as those of George Washington were and still are to American public school classrooms.

Such favorable images of the family doctor are all the more significant when one realizes how differently our current physicians are viewed by so many in our society. An abyss has opened up between many American doctors and their patients and, with the passage of every year, the gap seems to be growing wider and deeper, filled with elements of intolerable costs, greed, specialization and subspecialization, the insurance bureaucracy, managed care organizations, governmental inaction or ineffectiveness, and irresponsible legal opportunism, to name a few.

The types of physician idealized in the portraits of Fildes and Rockwell probably knew very little about the pathogenesis of the diseases with which they were confronted. They had few diagnostic tools at their command to enable them to make very precise diagnoses. And even if they had, there was very little available in the way of therapeutics to provide the cures they would have sought. Antibiotics, chemotherapy, hormonal replacement, advanced surgical techniques, and many other aspects of modern medicine we now take for granted were unknown to them. DNA, genetic engineering, and organ transplantation could hardly have been imagined by them.

The state of our grandparents' and great grandparents' health was precarious indeed. Life expectancy in the United States early in the twentieth century was only about fifty years for both men and women. Today, the rise as a group among us of those living twice as long hardly causes the bat of an eyelash. Childbirth during the bad old days was, in essence, a dangerous undertaking for any woman, and many did not survive it. Infants and young children were hardest hit of all. The great tenor Enrico Caruso was the first of only three children among the twenty-one his Neapolitan mother bore to survive beyond childhood, and this kind of experience was not exceptional elsewhere in Europe or the United States. A visit to any graveyard dating back to the early twentieth century, the late nineteenth century, and before, with all those tiny headstones, will provide ample evidence of this sad state of affairs.

The doctors who attempted to minister to the patients of these times, rich and poor alike, had nothing much to offer but prognostication. Keen observers of illness, they at least learned to predict who would live and who would die and did their best to provide comfort before the final, often dire outcome. Despite their limitations, they were, for the most part, looked upon with respect and admiration simply because *they were there* and because patients and their families knew *they cared.*

Human nature has not changed much, if at all, over the last hundred years. Our social institutions, however, have undergone enormous changes, and medical science has experienced an explosion of creativity and innovation. The combination of social evolution and scientific knowledge, overwhelmingly to the good, has paradoxically carried with it the baggage of an inefficient and suffocating morass that we now identify as our "health care system."

In reference to this, perhaps I should start out by stating what this book is *not.* This certainly is not a book about the current status of medical science; or the problems of medical economics; or questions of medical ethics. The effects of new knowledge on the rise of medical specialization and the fragmentation of medical care are common knowledge. The contradictory effects of the government's well-intentioned involvement in health care are well known to anyone with Medicare or Medicaid and their families. The uses and abuses of medical insurers are recognized by anyone who has ever filed a health-care claim. The intrusion of the legal profession and the so-called malpractice problem is constantly on the minds of most patients and all doctors. These and other issues concerning American medical care have been dealt with endlessly by countless experts within and without the profession, and the debates about the proper road to follow continue just as endlessly.

What this book does deal with is the way, after all the profound changes that have occurred in medical care over recent years, that doctors and patients view themselves and one another. Perhaps a better understanding of this will lead to a renewal of the feelings of trust and communication that seem to have been drained from the traditional doctor-patient relationship as depicted by Fildes, Rockwell, and other observers in the past. The method I have chosen is that of the storyteller. Through these vignettes I hope to make all who read this book, doctors and patients alike, come to a fuller realization that we are in this together.

A number of these stories involve the author, himself, sometimes thinly disguised. The remainder reflect the experiences of colleagues, patients, and friends who have been kind enough to share their experiences with me. The stories I tell are all true. Even the most fanciful tale, "A Man What Am," in which I have taken some literary license, is based on several physicians I have known.

Of all the ways to approach this subject perhaps the doctor-as-patient paradigm may be the most effective one. For this reason I have opened the book with the story of my own nearly fatal illness as a young man. The remaining tales were gleaned from more than fifty years as a medical student, house officer, internist, cardiologist, educator, medical investigator, and bedside physician.

I hope that for all who come to read these stories they will, in some way, allow each to understand the feelings and concerns of others a little better and—just as important—find greater understanding of themselves as well.

2

LANCE ARMSTRONG AND ME

AN EXERCISE IN DYING

The publication of the bicyclist Lance Armstrong's autobiography, *It's Not About the Bike,* and his description of the events surrounding the discovery of his testicular cancer in 1996 brought back to me memories of my own encounter with this disease about forty years earlier.

There were many similarities between young Armstrong at twenty-five and young Weisse at the same age. It was painful enlargement of the testicle that for both of us called attention to the disease. We both had experienced unusual tenderness of the breasts (gynecomastia) as the result of abnormal levels of circulating female hormones. We both were operated on for removal of the diseased testicle (orchiectomy) within a day of the diagnosis finally being made, and we both had highly malignant type tumors when the tissues were examined under the microscope. We were both very lucky; we lived to tell the tale.

However, there were also some striking differences between us. He was a world-class athlete and I, a medical student hitting the books, was relatively inactive physically. Armstrong engaged in considerable denial of his disease, while my problem was convincing my doctors, at first, of the peril I was in. Armstrong never really gave in to the disease, feeling all along that somehow he would conquer it. I was more focused on how to become resigned to my fate.

Finally, at the time of discovery, it turned out that Armstrong's cancer had spread (metastasized) to his lungs and brain, while my tumor, although suspected of having spread, turned out to be confined to the scrotum. Had this aspect of our respective cancers been reversed, Lance Armstrong would still have had the opportunity to write of his experiences. If, on the other hand, it was I who had had the metastases when my cancer was discovered in 1957, when the kind of chemotherapy that had saved Armstrong's life had not yet become available, I would not have survived to tell this story or any others in the succeeding years.

At one point in his book, Armstrong points out that everyone's encounter with illness is unique and exclusively his or her own. His experience with this disease, he claims, made him a better person; mine made me a better doctor.

As a medical educator responsible for the training of new physicians, I have always been interested in determining how to inject compassion into the medical curriculum. Of course, one cannot. Each individual will bring to his future practice of medicine only the sum total of his or her own individual experiences. It has long been a conviction of mine that only one who has previously endured the juggernaut of THE HOSPITAL—its baffling machinery; its unremitting regimentation; its phalanxes of physicians, nurses, technicians, aides, and others—only those who have endured and survived it can really relate to others who are passing through under their care at another time and another place. I have always thought of how nice it would be to have a magic wand with which I could make each of my students deathly ill in the hospital for only a week or so and then have them recover completely. Then I would be sure that for the rest of their lives they would empathize fully with their patients. Failing this, perhaps the story of my own illness might provide some kind of lesson for others, much in the way that Lance Armstrong's inspiring story has done for the general public.

During my extended confinement for testicular cancer in Brooklyn's Kings County Hospital when I was a senior medical student, I began a journal, continued for several weeks after my return home. It was kept a secret account, unknown to my parents, and its purpose was to explain to them the thoughts that occupied my mind during my acute illness and why I had chosen to spend what might have been the remaining few months of my life away from them. "To my parents. To be opened only after my death" was written on the envelope containing this document.

My parents never saw this journal. They are both dead and I am almost a fifty-year survivor. I hope it serves a somewhat different purpose now, conveying to the reader aspects of illness that do not appear in hospital charts. It lays bare the actions and reactions (some of them startling to me even now) of a young almost-physician under the severe stress of a life-threatening illness. In order to preserve the full flavor of the time, the place, and the person involved, this account of my illness is reproduced as originally written, rhetorical excesses and rough edges intact. It was, after all, a time when all kinds of extremes seemed merely appropriate.

HOSPITAL JOURNAL—September-October, 1957

It was in 1942 that Mr. and Mrs. Charles Weisse discovered as a result of a routine physical examination by the family doctor that their eleven-year-old son was less than physical perfection. In the course of his development, his right testicle had failed to descend normally from the abdominal cavity into the scrotum. A series of hormone injections followed, but "the high and the mighty" clung to its preferred position somewhere midway within the inguinal canal (groin). After some further consultation it was decided that an operation for the undescended testicle, with its associated congenital hernia, was to be performed.

Soon thereafter a Thorek procedure was carried out. This involved, among other manipulations, the temporary suturing of the recalcitrant testicle to the inner thigh by sutures passed through the skin of the thigh and through the wall of the scrotal sac into the substance of the testicle. After a few weeks of healing, the portion of the suture attaching the scrotum to the thigh was severed and the remaining scar tissue within the scrotum insured the fixation of the genital in the desired position.

The operation healed well except for occasional pains on

straining at the site of the incision. The testicle never lived up to expectations, however, remaining only two-thirds within the scrotum. It was hard, atrophic, and not very promising. Future physical examinations confirmed this, but inasmuch as its opposite blossomed and secondary male characteristics started to become increasingly evident, everyone seemed satisfied with the result. At this time I was about thirteen years of age. When I had reached the age of twenty, I experienced some pain in one of my breasts and felt a hardening of what I assumed to be glandular tissue within it. It was tender to palpation but there were no secretions and the symptoms disappeared spontaneously within a week's time. This recurred two or three times in the next seven years. * The last occurrence was five months prior to my present confinement. This episode was more alarming than the others inasmuch as both breasts were now involved simultaneously for the first time and the symptoms seemed more persistent than formerly.

By this time I was a third-year medical student at SUNY's (The State University of New York) Downstate Medical Center and the school in Brooklyn. I finally visited the Student Health Service, which was then being run by a rather self-important former student graduate and resident doctor at Long Island College Hospital and Kings County Hospital. In his short tenure in this post he had already established himself in the eyes of the students as not only unsympathetic but also cold, antagonistic, and belittling. When I expressed concern over the condition, he seemed to be of the opinion that, inasmuch as I was not a cirrhotic and could not, therefore, have an excess of estrogenic substances circulating in my blood as a result of liver

---

* This, in retrospect, should have raised suspicions. Although boys, during puberty, often experience pain in their breasts, when this occurs in a young man it suggests that abnormal female hormones are being produced, most likely from a malignant neoplasm.

failure, I had absolutely no business developing gynecomastia (swelling and/or tenderness of the breasts). The fact that I had a hard, partially undescended testicle I do not believe impressed him in the least. His course of treatment was of a tried and true variety. "Wait a month and if it still bothers you, come back."

During the next two weeks the trouble subsided and the succeeding two weeks concluded my third year of studies. Carefree and in high spirits, I embarked on a cross-continental motor trip with a classmate to investigate internships and take a course in medicine at the University of California in San Francisco. During the succeeding weeks it seemed to me that the abnormal right testicle had descended somewhat more into the scrotum and this pleased me. Perhaps some resumption of function was occurring. A year earlier at school, having read about the high incidence of testicular neoplasms in undescended testicles, I had shown my own specimen to a former student health doctor. He was considered an astute clinician and, although he thought the testicle atrophic and "not putting out many bullets," he assured me that, inasmuch as it was not located within the abdominal cavity or very high up in the inguinal canal, I had nothing to worry about. I happily—and unfortunately—had all doubts erased from my mind.

As the summer wore on I got the impression that my right testicle, which had always been smaller than my left, was beginning to approach it in size. At first I attributed this to the resumption of function at long last, but my wishful thinking gave way to genuine concern. My past experiences had always resulted in my discovery of a new phase of medical student hypochondriasis, and I hated to appear so foolish again in the light of past reassurances. Nevertheless, during the week that preceded the commencement of the new school year, I was determined to visit Student Health on the very first day of school. On that Friday night, two days before this, I was seized with a severe feeling of malaise and low back pain, especially on the right, which radiated to the right testicle. Rest in bed and cold applications caused subsidence of the back pain although the testicle remained tender.

I had the first appointment of the day with the Doubting Thomas in Student Health. He very definitely, at this time, indicated to me that he knew very little about enlarged testicles, but that he would make an appointment for me with the Urology Clinic when it might be convenient for them to see me in the next week or so. He turned the details over to his secretary. When, at my urging, she reached the attending urologist, Dr. Sidney Weinberg, on the telephone, I requested a word with him on a private extension. I gave him the briefest description of my past history and present illness. He requested that I await his arrival. An hour later he was examining me; two hours later I was admitted to Kings County Hospital for a diagnostic work-up and imminent surgery.

These rather precipitous developments were relayed to my family via telephone in as calm a manner as could be mustered. I then spent an hour in Dr. Weinberg's office awaiting his return from a conference. There, with a half-dozen different texts on urology to consult, I had myself quite a time adding to what meager knowledge I had already acquired regarding my complaint.

I learned that neoplasms of the testis constitute about 1 percent of all those occurring in males. Whenever there is any scrotal enlargement in the absence of trauma one should first note if it shows the typical cordlike anatomy of a varicocele (a network of engorged veins). If a mass transilluminates, with light passing through it from a source applied at one end, it might be a typical hydrocele, a collection of fluid rather than a solid cancer. One should see if it is limited to the epididymis (a tubal structure leading up from the testis) and suspect an inflammatory condition (epididymitis) especially if the mass is tender. In the absence of these findings, any scrotal swelling, especially if it is painless, hard, and heavy-feeling, should, without doubt, be considered a testicular neoplasm.

New growths of the testis are, like those in other locations, classified as either benign or malignant. The tendency for a new growth to spread helps to determine clinically what type of neoplasm is involved. Benign growths may gradually enlarge in size locally, but malignant ones aggressively invade surrounding tissue or spread to distant sites within the body (metastasize) via the blood stream or lymphatic channels. Given the reproductive type of tissue of which even normal testes are composed, it is not surprising that almost all testicular tumors turn out to be malignant. These tumors are classified according to cell type: seminomas, teratomas, embryonal and undifferentiated cell types of growth. The main trouble with all of these is that they often metastasize early and have perhaps gotten out of hand before they are called to the attention of a doctor. If the testis is intra-abdominal, then the patient is not even aware of when it begins enlarging. If they enlarge within the scrotum, lay people are often inclined to ignore them since most, at least in the early stages of the disease, are painless.

The age of incidence is in the sexual prime, usually between twenty and forty, with more than 40 percent of the cases first reaching the attention of an M.D. at this time. These tumors have a great variability to their behavior. The first symptoms may be caused by distant metastases. The most common site of spread are the lungs, where the metastases may grow silently for varying periods of time before causing symptoms, and the abdominal lymph nodes, where symptoms of pain (e.g. low back pain) may be caused by pressure of the enlarged nodes on adjacent structures. Gynecomastia may give a hint to the presence of one of these tumors since they may produce estrogenic

products. Incidence is forty to fifty times as great in undescended testes as compared with normally situated ones; they
occur more often on the right than the left; and, for some reason, doctors and medical students have constituted 10 percent
of the victims recorded in the past, probably due to their more
keen and wary appreciation of abnormal testicular changes.

In retrospect, it was evident that I was a classical case. I had
had an undescended testicle on the right. There was painless
enlargement of it until it formed a solid, heavy, nontranslucent
mass. I had experienced episodes of gynecomastia due to fluc-
tuating release of estrogens, and just prior to my confinement
for surgery, a spell of low back pain had occurred. My condition
became apparent at the age of twenty-five, and, last of all, Lord
help me, I was a medical student.

The prognosis depends on the presence and extent or spread
at the time of discovery and whether or not the tumor is sensitive to X-rays and therefore amenable to such therapy. Recur-
rences are most likely during the first year post-operatively after
orchiectomy (removal of the diseased testis). Even those tumors that seem limited to the testicle itself will recur elsewhere
in the body in 15 to 30 percent of patients during this time.
Following such a recurrence, survivals have varied from as little
as two years to as many as twenty years. As for myself, I only
hoped that the back pain I had experienced was due to spinal
nerve referable pain (sensory fibers from the scrotum entering
the spinal cord at the same level as those from the lower back
and therefore testicular pain actually being perceived as low
back pain) rather than actual lymph node involvement at that
level of the spine.

I felt like a caged tiger as I awaited the doctor in his office, but
at least had the presence of mind to acquire one of the few single rooms available on the surgical floors. Dr. Weinberg, when
he returned at last to have me admitted to the hospital, was very

sensibly noncommittal. When I confronted him with the overpowering evidence of my affliction, he replied, "It would be foolish for me to say anything at this time. We'll run a few tests tomorrow and on Wednesday we'll probably operate. Try not to worry about it."

Naturally he said the only thing possible under the circumstances, but I was hardly comforted. I reported to what might be my last official residence, seated myself on the high hospital bed fully clothed, and, for the first time in many years, I wept bitterly. I was terrified.

That same night I had an X-ray of my chest taken and this, fortunately, showed no evidence of metastases. The following morning I was taken to the radiology department for an IVP (intravenous pyelogram). This results in X-ray visualization of the ureters leading from the kidneys to the bladder. If there was any retroperitoneal involvement of the lymph nodes in the abdomen, these might displace the ureters from their normal course. Encouragingly, this did not seem to be the case, although on the official report there was a note stating that a couple of the films were missing.[*] Then, when I thought back on the low back pain I had experienced, I wondered if the lymph node involvement was actually present but not of a sufficiently great degree or in the proper location to cause a deviation of a ureter's course on the IVP. A twenty-four-hour urine collection was begun to analyze it for the presence of any possible abnormal female hormones, given my experiences of gynecomastia.

---

[*] Today such evidence of cancer spread could be obtained much more quickly, safely, and accurately with the use of a CT (computed tomography) scan.

The therapeutic program planned for me was as follows: first an orchiectomy, removing the diseased right testicle. If this was proved indeed to be cancerous after microscopic examination, I was to have a second operation to remove all lymph nodes draining the area running from the scrotum up into the abdominal region, the most likely first stopping place for testicular cancers. If the microscopic appearance of the cancer cells in the testicle indicated sensitivity to X-rays, then I would receive this treatment.

Following my brief emotional outburst on the night of admission, I regained my composure and since that time I guess I have kept on a pretty even keel. I always have been one to intellectualize situations, and this, without a doubt, was one helluva situation! Another forte has been my sense of humor and, thanks to my gene structure, I have been gifted with one improbable enough to seek the amusing aspects of even such a dreary and unpromising set of circumstances as those in which I found myself. I jotted off a, hopefully, reassuring letter to my older brother, suggesting to him that the whole family of idiomatic expressions dear to our generation of young males and including the term "balls" would, in my case, have to be changed to the singular. I signed it in a manner it would not take too much imagination to devise.

I took stock of my surroundings and began collecting amusing incongruities with which to barrage the train of concerned visitors that was certain to call on me. The basic ground plan of my room was a rectangle, with the door off-center at one end and a window at the other. One-quarter of the available space was occupied by my bathroom so that, as you entered, that portion was immediately on your left, the further half of the room opening up into an area which included a bed along the right wall, a bedside table, and a couple of metal chairs. A sink was in the far left corner, set off from the rest of the room by the tile backing on the wall immediately adjacent. As for the rest of the walls, they were painted in a sort of off-Department of Sanitation green and, in all probability, had not been retouched since the original application circa 1930. It reminded one of the scarred buildings of the Spanish Civil War, for some reason. Other furniture included a floor lamp that looked as if it had been borrowed from the grilling room of the Thirty-fourth Precinct Police Station, although I suspect it was just an ordinary hospital utility lamp. A tall stand that, in its younger days, served to hold intravenous fluid bottles now resembled some ingenious instrument of torture from the Tower of London and served to support my street clothes. The one gesture at adornment was a wall fan that insisted on circulating the air in but one remote corner of the room that I was never to occupy. This nevertheless proved somewhat helpful during the record-breaking heat wave that coincided with my hospital stay, and I was not deluding myself one bit—I was sitting very pretty as far as accommodations were concerned at Kings County Hospital.

After lunch on Tuesday I was visited by Dr. Hormel, the youthful and genial head of the Anesthesiology Department. He informed me that, inasmuch as there was no room to schedule the orchiectomy for the operating room on Wednesday, the operation would be performed by the eminent Dr. Hamm, head of the Urology Department, that very evening at 5 p.m. We agreed on spinal anesthesia—Hormel because he thought it least likely to result in any complications; I because I wanted to be in on everything that transpired during the course of the operation. I figured this was worth the risk of the post-operative headache that sometimes occurs with this type of anesthesia. When the time came I downed my three grains of Seconal and submitted my arm for a dose of morphine to top off the pre-anesthetic medication. Needless to say, as I was wheeled into the operating room I was feeling no pain, and, as it turned out, Dr. Weinberg would be performing the surgery after all. (Frankly, at this point I would not have been able to tell if it were Tonto and the Lone Ranger.)

I remember Dr. Hormel administering the spinal and the hot and prickly feeling that I sensed in my lower extremities shortly thereafter as I lost the ability to move them. Before I knew it, they had made the initial incision of which I was not even conscious. I felt only slightly dull slaps, which I interpreted as the clamping off of bleeders. At about this time Dr. Hormel "pulled a fast one" on me, allowing some pentothal, a rapidly acting barbiturate, to flow into my IV, and I drifted off to dreamland. My next few memories were that of being lifted into the recovery room bed; then being catheterized for urine; then the following day gazing into the bright features of the student nurse assigned to me; and then the figure of Dr. Hormel hovering over my bedside the first couple of post-operative days to assure me that all that talk of post-spinal anesthesia headache was merely Communist propaganda. Except for a few gas pains, my recovery from the operation was uneventful. I voided spontaneously the first post-op day and was soon walking about freely.

These first days passed by with ease, what with the business of eating, washing, walking, antibiotic injections, and having my pulse and temperature taken periodically. My father was with me almost constantly in the afternoons even after I no longer needed his assistance. I allowed him the luxury of waiting on me hand and foot to relieve himself, in part, of the great worry that was bearing on him. I have tried sincerely to shield the absolute truth from him and the rest of the family, but this has been difficult as I have never been a good liar and my face more than once has been described as "an open book."

As for my own morale, it has been boosted most successfully by Mike Matson, an old friend of the family who left a very lucrative general dentistry practice in upstate New York to study oral surgery in Brooklyn. At present he is serving as chief resident of that department at Kings County Hospital. He is a big, gruff man, about forty, with an open way about him and an indefinable knack for making even a wiseacre like me think that he knows all that there is to know about the whole business and still is not the least bit worried about ultimately a good outcome. My classmates were also a balm to my somewhat frayed nerves. They told me I was not missing a thing in Environmental Medicine, the current rotation, and let me out of my own life for a few moments to share their daily activities, which were and, I suppose for a time anyway, will be mine once I emerge from here.

Dr. Weinberg, to whom I owe a great deal, has been at times somewhat puzzling to me, but I attribute this to my own state of mind rather than any failings on his part. He certainly has not the most enviable task in the world, that of treating a fairly advanced medical student with a disease of notoriously poor prognosis. I assume there is little else he can do but say nice things until the final showdown. The first of these involved the pathology report on the specimen removed at operation (the right testicle). The report was due on the Friday following my surgery, and I spent the longest morning of my life awaiting his arrival, even though I knew beforehand in my heart how it must read. Dr. Weinberg is a bouncy, cheerful-looking man in his forties; on the chubby side with red, wavy hair receding from his crown and freckles scattered over his usually radiant countenance. He breezed in with two cardboard boxes under one arm. From one of these he withdrew a looseleaf-bound black text, which he introduced as the new textbook on urology that he and Dr. Hamm had coauthored. It was quite handsome and, as I leafed through, attempting to appear as if there was nothing else in the world on my mind, he informed me in a sort of verbal postscript that the Pathology Department was still studying the sections in order to be quite sure that the report would be ready the following Monday. Interpreted, this meant that they simply had not gotten around to it, but I muttered something appropriately cooperative-sounding and he dashed out to deliver the shiny texts to their future owners. I sat back for a long weekend at this Goliath of all city hospitals.

A few feet away, to the left of my room on the second floor of Building A, is an open walk paved in brown tile and leading to Building B. Inasmuch as no entrance from Building B seems to enter out on the walk, this space assumes the title of Ward A-12 Sun Porch. In truth, you could hardly speculate that this area, some thirty feet in width and one hundred yards long, was actually devised for the recreation of the patients. As one enters out on it, he hurries past the first few feet adjacent to the side of the building in order to avoid any of the sputum specimens descending from a host of possibly active tuberculars on the floors above. Now there is a choice of either balustrade lining the walk. The one on the right is not too promising: a few feet below is barren concrete extending to more dull red brick for eleven stories more of A-B building. The left balustrade, on the contrary, offers unrivaled vistas for exploration if one will only apply himself. Directly below one sees the heart of one of this institution's key operations, the garbage disposal platform, and countless hours are spent watching the gay, spirited revelry of the garbage men as they load to the brim the large metal units lined up along the platform before they are carted away by the Department of Sanitation.

Across the way is the latest aesthetic accomplishment of the city planning board, a four-story edifice of granite and black marble that houses the Morgue and Department of Pathology. It sort of gives patients something to look forward to after the rather drab architectural surroundings on this side of paradise.

As one gazes up into that part of the blue not claimed by soaring city masonry, he notices droves of friendly feathered creatures looking indulgently down upon the whole pastoral scene. They are called pigeons by most of the others, but I know them to be vultures in disguise and cannot help but feel like some bit of carrion awaiting future disposal. Frankly, it is rather difficult to decide what the function of these flighty creatures might really be. Following our traditional Sunday chicken dinner, the population, as I later once again gazed upward, seemed curiously decimated.

Dr. Weinberg did not arrive on Monday with the pathological report until 6 p.m. Inasmuch as I had been expecting him at about 1:30 at the latest, I was literally seething with anxiety as I attempted to pass the unyielding hours comfortably by playing cards with my father. The news was not good. The neoplasm was of the embryonal variety, i.e. resistant to radiotherapy. Although there was no evidence of it having spread, they were playing it safe. Dr. Jesse Richardson from St. Albans Naval Hospital had been contacted and, in order to be sure that if there was any spread to the lymph nodes on the right that had escaped radiological detection, the removal of the whole chain of lymph nodes on the right (all along the course of the aorta and spine in the posterior portion of the abdomen) would be undertaken. If the cancer was found to have invaded any of those nodes, a similar procedure would be performed on the left inasmuch as there is some communication between the lymph drainage between the two sides.

My father remained and took the news fairly well at first, although later we both broke up over it. I now am in a hurry to get all this over with inasmuch as only surgical exploration and subsequent pathological sections will ascertain whether or not there has been a spread of the neoplasm. If these prove negative, then I can rest relatively easy. If the nodes are positive, then I can at least sustain the hope that such a spread has been cut off at its first stage. So round two is coming up . . .

My emotional reaction to this sorry state of affairs was first fear, then anger, then sadness, then resignation, then hope dominating at last with remnants of the others still in evidence.

The fear mainly preceded the precipitous series of events on the day before my first operation, culminating in my sobbing it out alone in my room, hopeless and devoid of spirit. When I was able to recover from the initial shock of it all, I mustered whatever ego reserve I had left and fought these battles myself at night when the thoughts and events of the past day tend to distill themselves in one's consciousness. The first night after the operation I looked heavenward and cried under my breath, "F—k you God. F—k you. F—k, f—k, f—k you." I turned my fist to the wall, punctuating each blow with other expletives under my breath. But it takes too much energy to stay angry very long at a God you do not believe in, not even this close to death. Anger gave way to sadness. I had not had too easy a time of it as I looked back on my life; all that I had gained thus far had come the hard way, especially medical school. Now that I was finally to graduate, I had been stricken with an almost surely fatal disease. I, who love children and looked forward to the day when I might gaze fondly on my family about me, would have to look forward now to a solitary and sharply curtailed existence.

At times like these one thinks of God and Death and little else. For the first time, I must confess disbelief and maintain my agnosticism in the face of our real ignorance in the matter. I have no answers and no arguments. I cannot honestly accept this concept of a supreme being as it exists for believers of any faith even though, by so doing, I acknowledge with my demise the totality of death and the nonexistence of a hereafter. I am not afraid of death, although I dislike it intensely. Life's pleasures are many, and I, for one, appreciated them to the full. I hate the thought of partaking of them no more, of being no more. I hate it now because I am young and the world holds promise for me. Perhaps if I were old and could look back on the full course of my life, the prospect of dying would not be quite so detestable.

You may reckon that this attitude is braggadocio, that everyone fears death. Most people fear it because it is the unknown and the circumstances surrounding it are usually painful and terrifying to consider. To me, death is not wholly a stranger. The little clinical experience I have had has robbed it of its uniqueness if not its mystery. As for the circumstances surrounding death that strike fear in peoples' hearts, despite the setting, they are often most concerned with the experiencing of pain. I am convinced that the prolonged demise of any dear one is much harder for his family than for himself, and is a strong argument for euthanasia. The agony prolonged is not experienced by the occupant of the deathbed, numbed to pain either by his own failing condition or the medications of his physician. It is felt by that inner circle of his family that waits outside the door and dies a little with him with the passing of each added, senseless day leading to the inevitable.

At present I vacillate between utter resignation to a sealed doom and almost unconscious prayer to the God I so glibly denied. When I consider the limited time left me, I contemplate various plans I might make to spend my final days as enjoyably as possible. A trip to Europe is one consideration, for example, before I enter a terminal phase and hospital confinement. At present, the dread prospect of spending all the rest of my very few days as a surgical specimen looms menacingly before me. All this will have to await the outcome of the next few weeks' surgery. Fingers crossed.

I would like to prove an exception to the knowing prognostications of the urological texts. The one saving grace of our very incomplete knowledge of medicine is that it gives one a chance to hope. I am sort of a nice fellow and would probably live a very good kind of life on earth. I most assuredly would have done some good for many people. This is the personal tragedy involved. This and the realization that the main hope for fulfillment that my parents once had now flickers before them on the brink of eternity. They have had a rather lousy life, all things considered, and I, perhaps, might have been one of the redeeming features. This is a cruel trick to play on them, whether it is God, Providence, or the Three Fates dealing the cards. I almost want to live more for their happiness and peace of mind than my own. I end with a hope for as much time to breathe in the wonderful world about me as possible. I have discovered it at last, I hope not too late.

Two weeks later:

I am writing what I hope will be the final section of this personal record in the relative quiet and security of my own room at home.

What Dr. Weinberg had kindly described to my parents as a "minor procedure" involved the stripping of all the retroperitoneal lymph nodes alongside the aorta from its course in the chest to the pelvic region where it splits into the two common iliac arteries. I suspected this would be a rather tedious procedure and advised my parents that it would probably take a number of hours.

Early that Thursday morning of September 19, 1957, my sleep was interrupted by the administration of preoperative sedatives, and I was hardly conscious of being transported to the operating room a few hours later. Thus I was never able to greet my benefactor, Captain Richardson, who, I believe, had performed about seventy of these procedures before on other young men and, indeed, was one of those to devise the procedure in the first place.

My first recollection of the day was that of being in the recovery room immediately post-operatively and looking up into Dr. Weinberg's smiling face. The operation, which he had expected to last six or seven hours, had gone exceptionally well. The entire procedure had taken three and a half hours, and none of the nodes removed had appeared grossly to be involved. These were the first optimistic words I had heard from the good doctor since the beginning of all this, and before I lapsed into unconsciousness again I felt somewhat reassured.

The surgical incision extended from the lower border of the right shoulder blade (scapula) across the rib cage where the tenth rib was removed to permit access to the nodes at that level, down the lateral part of the abdomen, and across the inguinal region to the scrotum. This permitted the removal of all lymph nodes immediately draining the scrotal area where the neoplasm had originated. Thus, should there have been metastases prior to the first operation, this would cut off any spread presumably at the first stopping place. The fact that there seemed to be no involvement of these nodes was indeed encouraging and explained the lower back pain I had experienced on the basis of referred pain from the scrotum and not enlarged lymph nodes in the abdominal area pressing on adjacent nerve fibers as I had feared.

The next three days were to prove the most painful that I have ever endured. The original order for narcotics was for 50 mgm of Demerol (a morphine substitute) every four hours, but I found that I was metabolizing it at such a rapid rate that the effect had worn off completely within an hour or so. As a result, for the first twenty-four hours post-op, before I could get the order changed I spent three of every four hours in unrelieved pain. Following this the dosage was boosted to 75 mgm every three hours, which was quite a relief although I ordered the nurse myself to reduce the dose to 50 mgm or even skipped an injection when I felt I could stick it out. I had enough troubles without adding narcotic addiction to them.[*]

As I lay there moaning and groaning and awaiting the next blessed needle, I found myself categorizing the different varieties of pain I was experiencing and the way the Demerol seemed to attack one type, then another, in order of their increasing severity. The most minor of my complaints involved the constant backache from so many days in bed, along with swollen buttocks and arms from the multiplicity of injections I had been receiving ever since my first operation. Then there was the sharp right chest pain where the rib had been removed, which I felt with every inspiration, and the right shoulder pain referred from areas of the diaphragm irritated during the course of the second operation. Finally there was the persistent

---

[*] Times have not changed. Recent studies have repeatedly indicated that physicians and surgeons, without justification, routinely prescribe inadequate doses of pain-relieving medication for their patients in need of such relief.

dull ache of the incision, aggravated by any pressure or muscular contraction, especially on coughing up secretions periodically.

Following the intramuscular administration of the drug, within five minutes I would find myself still conscious of the pain but not minding it so much. I would feel a slight sensation of vertigo as the full effects became manifest, and suddenly the dull ache at the back of my spine was gone. Following this, the soreness of the injections disappeared; then the chest pain, and finally all of the wound pain. A feeling of warmth and euphoria enveloped me and at last the longed for comfort of sleep. Later on during my recovery, when I was actually pain free, I again had Demerol administered in order to see if the effects would be duplicated, but found that without the stimulus of really severe pain the effects of the drug were minimal. Codeine, likewise, proved practically without effect at this point.

Post-operatively my academic curiosity regarding the experiencing of the various procedures I had, myself, performed on patients, was more than amply satisfied. I received my first blood transfusion (three pints: two during and one following surgery) and was surprised to find how chilling was the effect of administered refrigerated blood. I had intravenous solutions administered to me for two days after surgery and learned how uncomfortable even a properly inserted intravenous needle can be after twenty-four or forty-eight hours. To prevent gaseous distention of my inactive digestive tract (partly caused by the narcotics) I received numerous Harrison irrigations rectally to remove gas from my colon. At one point the resident urologist feared that too much gas was accumulating in my stomach and passed a Levin tube through my nose, down my throat, and into my stomach to decompress it. This was undoubtedly the purest agony I have ever experienced. Ordinarily there is some retching due to a gagging reflex during such insertions but in this instance, with every gag the attendant abdominal contractions resulted in a series of excruciating spasms along the course of the suture line that left me breathless, the tears of pain flowing from my eyes at the completion of the maneuver. The manner of my distress was unnerving even to the experienced resident, and I could detect the apprehension in his eyes. The Levin tube remained in place for thirty-six hours and gave the sensation of a sore throat with swallowing. I was also fed liquids through the tube, which felt queer but not unpleasant.

The introduction of the Levin tube led, in a few hours, to a situation that drove me frantic. From my left nostril it was hooked up by a very short rubber extension tube to a suction machine for the removal of any gas swallowed. At the same time, the irritation of the Levin tube in my throat led to an increased amount of bronchial secretions that had to be coughed up. In order to get these secretions up, I had to assume a postural drainage position on my left side. However, the suction machine to which the stomach tube was connected could only be fitted in to the right side of my bed and the tubing was so short that I could not bring my head to a dependent position in order to expectorate without pulling on the tube. Each time I did this, however, the tube pressed against a very sensitive nerve in the septum of my nose causing extreme discomfort. One can imagine how distracted I became in my debilitated state, but fortunately this did not go on too long before one of my classmates dropped in and helped to rig up a longer connection to the suction apparatus. Providentially Dr. Weinberg arrived the next day and removed the tube entirely. I shall never fail to "feel for" any future postsurgical patients that happen to fall under my charge!

Early ambulation following surgery has become the common practice in this country in recent years. While assigned to the surgical wards last year, I shivered as aged patients, following subtotal gastrectomies, cholecystectomies, and other major procedures were routed out of bed and literally tongue-whipped by their attendants to walk up and down the halls one or two days post-operatively. In my own case, as little inclined as I felt to skip down the halls, the beneficial effects of ambulation on the first post-operative day were readily apparent. The act of having risen from bed and taken at least a few faltering steps seemed to accelerate the entire recuperative process.

During the first three post-operative days I literally abhorred the visitations of all well-wishers, oddly enough, especially those dearest to me, my parents. It was bad enough to be in pain but having to fear evincing any evidence of it was an added burden I could not endure. So it was I who drove my family from the bedside; and as for the rest of the visitors, waved, then waved them off as well. This reinforced my convictions about visits to postsurgical patients, and I resolved to bar all visitors if and when the Richardson procedure was performed on my left side.

The urology resident, a fireballing young man from the Philippines, was kind enough to arrange to have special nurses assigned to me during these hard times, and I certainly did not lack for excellent attention. From 8 a.m. until midnight I was assigned to pretty, cheerful, and efficient student nurses. At midnight a saint by the name of Mrs. Mary Grogan arrived on the scene to contribute her thirty-two years of experience in nursing and a lifetime experience in consideration, kindness, and humanity to getting me through the rough nights.

As I gained ground, my thoughts shifted from my immediate distress to future problems I would have to face. Dr. Weinberg again awaited pathological reports, this time on the chain of lymph nodes removed. He told me that they appeared free of disease at surgery, and, if microscopic examination confirmed this, it would not be necessary to undergo the operation of lymph node stripping on my left side. The days and nights dragged on. Thursday, a week from the date of the operation, came, and still there was no news. Thursday and Friday were the holidays of the Jewish New Year and Dr. Weinberg was not in the hospital. I hoped to see him Saturday, but he did not appear. Sunday morning, following a hint from the resident the night before, I advised my parents over the telephone to bring a topcoat just in case. Dr. Weinberg arrived with the news that the pathological specimens were negative for tumor and I could go home that day.

It is good to be home and among one's own again. Each day brings just a little more strength and a little less pain. As far as anyone knows, I am well again with nothing more to show for my ordeal than the operative scar, which I refer to alternately as my personal plan of the Trans-Siberian Railroad and Route 17 to the Catskills on a Friday night in July.

The prognosis remains in doubt. In the past, as I have indicated before, patients such as I did not have much to hope for, but this was before the institution of such radical surgery as I have undergone. The statistical results of these innovations have yet to be published, but thus far they seem to be achieving a good deal more in the way of results than the possibly inadequate surgery of the past. Dr. Weinberg seems to believe that if I get through the next two years without trouble he will no longer be worried.

As for my state of mind, I might say that I initially may have been somewhat pessimistic. Now I am just hoping to myself that I am one of the lucky ones that go into the compilation of the statistics. In view of the guarded prognosis, I realize that I must make certain adjustments in my personal life.

For one thing, I must do my best to avoid any deep emotional involvement. I certainly do not want to be instrumental in latching some sweet young thing on to a very potential corpse—which is what I will be for the next two years at least. At the end of this time, if I am still free of complaints, being of sound mind and body, I will feel free to dispose any woman in question to a greatly decreased risk.

Another consideration is that of my career plans. I am more determined than ever to leave New York. When I arrive on the new scene I will be able to apprise the local urologists of my problem and have them follow me. If I do go in for some more surgery, regardless of its efficacy, I certainly do not wish to submit my family again to the strain that this will certainly involve. I would even be inclined to keep any such future procedures completely hidden from them. Only if I enter some terminal phase would I wish them to know of it and be able to see me only at the very last, thus saving them—and me as well—a great deal of useless anxiety and heartache. Should such a sorry state of affairs ever come about I will see to it that they receive this record posthumously in order to understand my actions.

I realize that all of this will seem rather calculated and somewhat pessimistic, but I have never been one to let loose ends lie about, and certainly in an affair as important as this I wish to have everything in order.

Now one starts to live again and tries to think of only the good things that the future might bring.

October 3, 1957

POSTSCRIPT

After some weeks at home I returned to my studies. I was given credit for the clerkship I had taken in California the summer preceding my illness and was thus able to graduate with my class in June 1958. Outwardly my existence seemed, once more, to assume a normal course, but in reality it was peppered with aberrations and inconsistencies.

On the day of my return to our apartment in midtown New York, my mother prepared for me a grand meal featuring my favorite, veal parmigiana. Unaccustomed to such spicy food after weeks on a bland hospital diet, I developed stomach cramps after the meal and immediately interpreted this as evidence of cancer spread rather than a very obvious case of dyspepsia.

A few weeks after my return to medical school, by some subterfuge, without identifying myself, I managed to obtain temporary possession of the slides of the lymph nodes that had been removed at the second operation. I wanted to see them for myself, suspecting that I had been lied to in order to protect my feelings. My first scan of the slides convinced me that I was correct. Under the microscope I saw cells with large, darkly staining nuclei that I immediately "recognized" as cancer cells. Later I learned that they were simply innocent nerve cells that had been adjacent to the lymph nodes and removed along with them.

Dr. Weinberg had cautioned me against contemplating marriage for at least the two years it would take to determine with some degree of assurance whether or not they had overlooked any metastases. After one year had passed I manufactured a fake fiancée to test him. The advice remained firm. In the meantime I made monthly visits to the cancer clinic at Memorial Hospital in New York where periodic blood samples were drawn to measure hormone levels that might signal a recurrence of the disease. Despite our knowledge of the advances made in cancer therapy, the eeriness of that sensation, sitting among "the doomed" in the waiting room, was and is indescribable.

The X-ray resistance to the type of cell that characterized my tumor and which was a cause for initial disappointment proved to be a blessing in disguise. If the histology had indicated radiosensitivity, I probably would have received massive radiation to the lower abdomen, which may have prevented my siring the two angels that became the joy of my existence. Now adults, my daughter is a high school English teacher and, as of this writing, is preparing to present us with our first grandchild. Our son is an academic veterinary surgeon and assistant professor at the University of Pennsylvania. My partner in all this, my wife, Laura, and I married in 1967 almost ten years after this story began.

Following my graduation from Downstate I took an internship in San Francisco at Mount Zion Hospital for the reasons stated above but, for years afterward, on an annual basis I continued dropping Christmas cards to the "score keeper" at Memorial in New York, letting her know simply that I was alive and symptom-free. It was something special, being a good statistic; and after ten years of reporting I was relieved of this responsibility and declared cured.

As we made ward rounds at the San Francisco Veterans Administration Hospital, where I had begun my residency in internal medicine following the year at Mt. Zion, I assisted in the care of a number of youngish men with testicular cancer. Not surprising was the frequency of this, given the patient populations at such hospitals. The attending physician would often present me to some poor young man with hopelessly disseminated testicular cancer and try to hold out hope for him.

"Look at Dr. Weisse here. He had the same thing you have and he's doing fine!"

I trust it gave some comfort to the patient, but it did little to boost my own morale. I carried with me the knowledge that, timewise, I was still not out of the woods, statistically speaking. I also carried with me the knowledge that those who have had cancer in one testicle stand as much as a tenfold increased incidence in the opposite testicle when compared to the general population. I also knew that if the tumor suddenly appeared in the abdominal nodes or in my lungs I was a goner. Chemotherapy was only in its relative infancy in those days, and even with more powerful agents available today the chance of a cure for a metastatic embryonal carcinoma of the testis is only about 50 percent. If the brain or liver is involved it is far worse.

Years later my closest friend and classmate confided to me that, following the surgery, he awaited the emergence of Dr. Weinberg from the operating suites for the verdict. The urologist had said nothing but simply responded with a thumbs down gesture. I guess his cheerful dissembling was quite an accomplished performance after all. When I attend class reunions now every five years or so, I see more than just the glint of recognition in the eyes of my classmates. There is also relief and elation ("Look, he beat the odds. That's great!"). Some of them have approached me in recent times and asked how, immediately after that hospitalization, I could have calmly taken up where I had left off and continued to function so well. The value of routine, of daily chores and responsibilities, is that they serve as a rock of normalcy in a sea of uncertainty for the cancer patient.

Five years after my own surgery I was doing a fellowship in cardiovascular research in Salt Lake City at the University of Utah School of Medicine. One of the medical students developed testicular cancer in his junior year. At the time of the discovery it had already spread to his lungs. Still under chemotherapy and intermittent radiation treatments, he resumed his studies following an initial hospitalization and poor response to treatment. He died in the middle of his senior year. Many wondered at his ability to go on in the manner he did. I understood perfectly.

Dr. Weinberg exchanged the gray steel and concrete of Brooklyn for the prevailing verdure of the Virgin Islands, where he continued his practice for many years. Dr. Hamm retired to upper New York State. I lost track of Dr. Hormel, the kindly anesthesiologist who attended my surgery; and, sad to say, I never had the opportunity of meeting to thank in person Dr. Jesse Richardson, whose efforts meant so much to my later life and happiness.

3

THE CROCK

AN OLD PATIENT TEACHES A
YOUNG DOCTOR A FATAL LESSON

Crock n. 1: any piece of crockery, as a jar, esp. of coarse earthen-ware. 2: Scot. and dialectal Eng. An old or barren ewe.

—Webster's New Collegiate Dictionary

Crock n.: A patient with symptoms that are poorly defined, not supported by objective evidence either on physical or laboratory examination, difficult if not impossible to alleviate, and provocative of extreme frustration and hostility from doctors called upon to provide treatment.

—Medical lore, unpublished

The year was 1960, when many modern medical innovations, such as intensive care units, were just about ready to be introduced and interns like Butler often "flew by the seats of their pants."

Butler looked up at the wall clock as he hung up the telephone. It was 3:15 in the morning. "Jee-sus," he muttered, "This is going to be another one of those nights."

He had already admitted to his service a young girl in diabetic coma, and she was not responding well to his treatment. The elderly man with bilateral pneumonia looked as if he were going into respiratory failure. And the alcoholic who had entered the hospital with delirium tremens had just vomited up blood. Now a "possible coronary" was on his way up on the elevator from the emergency room.

"That coronary has just arrived on the floor, Dr. Butler . . ."

"OK, Mrs. Winston," he replied to the floor nurse. "I'll check him over right now, but I'd like you to call the lab and get me the results on the electrolytes and blood sugar I drew on that diabetic girl. And you better have our shaky friend who just vomited typed and cross-matched for six units of blood. He may need them before the night is over. And put him on vital signs each half hour times four and then every hour until we see which way he is going."

As the night nurse went about her duties, the intern turned his attention to his latest admission, an agitated, balding white man who appeared to be in his mid-fifties.

"What seems to be the trouble, Mr. . . . uh," he glanced at the admitting slip, ". . . Mr. Goodfriend?"

"What's the matter, you ask! I may be dying. I have this heart condition. All my life I've had heart trouble. Call my doctor, Dr. Gold. He'll tell you. He takes care of me for all my medical problems."

"I meant, what are you feeling? Are you in pain?"

Actually, aside from anxiety, outwardly the man looked to be in pretty good health to Butler. His color was good; his breathing did not seem to be labored.

"It's the pain in my chest that's killing me. That's what my dear ex-wife would like, but I won't give her the satisfaction. I'll live to see her in *her* grave first. Just to spite her, I'll . . ."

"Well, let me check you over, Mr. Goodfriend."

The patient's vital signs—his blood pressure, pulse and respiratory rates, and body temperature—were normal. The skin was normally warm and without excessive sweating. There was no evidence of heart failure as might have been indicated by engorgement of the neck veins or the sound of fluid in the lungs as the intern listened with his stethoscope over various parts of the chest. The heart itself sounded unremarkable: there was a regular rhythm without any abnormal sounds or murmurs. The abdomen and extremities were similarly unrevealing of pathology.

Throughout the physical examination, the excitable Mr. Goodfriend kept up a constant babble about his problems with his wife, his disagreements with his business partner, his battles with his accountant, his distrust of lawyers, etc. Butler soon learned from his patient that not only had the internist, Dr. Gold, been kept on hand for medical problems, but also that a psychiatrist had been the overseer of Mr. Goodfriend's emotional problems and had been managing his various neuroses for at least five years.

Butler placed a call to Dr. Gold to get the essential facts about Mr. Goodfriend's past medical history, but Dr. Gold was on vacation and his partner was on his way to another hospital on an emergency call.

An electrocardiogram was taken by Butler, himself. It appeared to be totally within normal limits. He temporized by ordering a sedative for Mr. Goodfriend and turned his attention once again to the other patients with whom he had been preoccupied earlier in the evening. He learned that the blood sugar level of the diabetic girl was not lowering toward normal, as it should have following his treatment with insulin. Perhaps she was insulin-resistant. The alcoholic had vomited another cup of blood. The color of the patient with pneumonia was beginning to take on a disturbingly bluish cast.

By the time Butler's backup, the medical resident, arrived, he found his intern fuming.

"Gottfried, those bastards in the ER are having an acute case of the Dumping Syndrome with me again. Every crock that walks in seems to wind up on my floor. I've already got my hands full with three very sick patients. I don't have time to waste on a cardiac neurotic."

Dr. Gottfried, although only a year or two older than Butler, rose to the challenge and assumed the role of the senior seasoned physician for the benefit of his subordinate. "Now, now Butler, I know you've had a bad night, but you should not let it affect your judgment. A physician must not only treat diabetic coma and pneumonia but also the emotional ills to which his patient might be prey. And who knows? Your Mistuh Goodfriend might have a heap'a heart trouble after all. Now, how 'bout mah takin' a look at him with ya, Doctuh?"

Whenever Gottfried began his unctuous sermonizing to an intern or patient, his voice took on the twang of what might barely pass for that of a Texas Ranger. He obviously believed that this ploy increased his effectiveness of delivery, but it was a curious tactic for a five-and-a-half-foot, moon-faced young man from Brooklyn.

Butler stared ahead, expressionless during the harangue. "Christ," he thought to himself, "he's playing Gary Cooper again!"

The two house physicians approached the bedside of the new patient, who had been installed in a private room. No sooner did Gottfried begin an inquiry about the patient's symptoms than he received a psychic barrage of invectives, as had his junior partner shortly before.

"Fine, fine. Ah think ah get the picture. Now let me just check you ovah a bit, Mr. Goodfriend."

The resident conscientiously checked all the pertinent negatives of the examination that Butler had previously reported to him. His findings were identical to those of his intern. At one point, he had the patient sit up and dangle his legs over the side of the bed so that he might go to the other side and, standing behind Mr. Goodfriend, he listened at the bases of the lungs with his stethoscope. As he did so and was assured that the lung findings were, indeed, totally normal, he glanced over the patient's shoulder at Butler and winked slyly.

"Mistuh Goodfriend," Gottfried pontificated, "we think you are goin' to do just fine, but we are goin' to watch you heah a few days. We have every expectation that you will be goin' home soon in as fine a fettle as evah."

"Oh thank you, doctor, both of you. I knew I could count on you. You've been wonderful to me!"

With this Goodfriend suddenly grasped Gottfried's hand and

kissed it. The resident, mortified, turned crimson as he tried to extricate himself. Meanwhile Butler looked heavenward in exasperation and turned toward the door of the room. He was soon followed into the hall by Gottfried, who had rapidly regained his composure. He placed a fatherly hand on Butler's shoulder and once again launched into his "Understanding Physician" routine.

Suddenly, they heard the sound of a severe coughing spell coming from Goodfriend's room and rushed back in. Goodfriend was on his knees at the foot of the bed facing the door and grasping the bed board tightly with both hands. He was terrified and ashen in color as large amounts of blood-tinged frothy sputum came pouring out of his mouth and on to the floor and bedclothes. He was in acute pulmonary edema, literally drowning in his own secretions.

Butler called down the hall for the nurse to bring the emergency medication tray as he and Gottfried tied lengths of rubber tubing around the patient's thighs to reduce the amount of blood returning to the failing heart, from which fluid was backing up into the lungs. They attempted to reassure Goodfriend as they worked on him and placed an oxygen mask over his face. Panic-stricken and fighting for his breath, the desperate patient threw off the mask as his wheezing and gurgling became more audible and more pink froth poured out of his mouth and nose at an alarming rate.

The nurse was soon on the scene and drew up some morphine to treat the attack, but by now the patient was thrashing about wildly and uncontrollably. They could not get him to hold still while they attempted to administer the medication. Finally, in desperation, both physicians straddled him and Butler struggled with an arm to find a vein through which he could administer the morphine. Several times he had just entered one with the needle only to have the arm abruptly jerked away from him. Finally he succeeded and began to infuse the drug slowly. Suddenly the struggling stopped and the patient was quite still. He was dead. The entire attack and the efforts to control it could not have lasted more than a few minutes.

A long-distance call to Dr. Gold turned up the fact that Mr. Goodfriend had been a cardiac neurotic all his adult life. In later years he did have some justification for this, however. A victim of coronary heart disease, he had suffered his first massive heart attack five years earlier and had had two additional "coronaries" since that time. The normalization of the electrocardiogram, one or two years following a heart attack, was not an unusually rare occurrence, nor was the absence of physical findings during a new episode. The admission that night to Butler's service had undoubtedly represented the final attack for the unfortunate man.

When the night of the Goodfriend episode had come to a close, Butler was the first in the hospital cafeteria during the early morning hours. He would take a quick breakfast before going to his quarters for a shower and then return to his floor for morning rounds.

He mused over the occurrences of the previous night. The diabetic girl was not resistant to insulin after all and was now fully awake. The alcoholic patient had no further vomiting of blood and would have a GI series that morning to look for an ulcer. The man with pneumonia had been placed on a breathing apparatus and intermittent oxygen. He was "pinking up" nicely.

And Mr. Goodfriend? The young doctor wryly admitted to himself that perhaps he had been premature in his judgments, that perhaps he had allowed himself too easily to consider little else in the crock but the obvious crack.

4

DEVOTION

SOMETIMES IT'S HARD TO LET GO; OTHER TIMES . . .

Fathers' Day and Mothers' Day were always sure to be busy ones at the psychiatric observation unit of Brooklyn's Kings County Hospital. They were the two days of the year that many of the "kids" arranged to see their elderly parents and often-times the annual visitation revealed that either Mom or Dad was not "hitting on all cylinders" anymore. Only one thing to do, naturally: off with them to the State Hospital, then and now the poor man's Leisure Village. Before committal to the state hospital could be made, however, a short period of observation at Kings County was necessary. Then an abbreviated legal hearing on the premises enabled transfer to the neighboring state institution.

Not all family calls to the Admitting Unit were as brutally matter-of-fact as the foregoing might suggest. On one particular Fathers' Day there was the saddening spectacle of the guilt-ridden daughter who had been caring for her senile father and had been coerced by other members of the family to have him committed to the state hospital. This haggard housewife, in her thirties, had been caring for him in her home along with four small children and without any assistance from other family members. She was clearly crumbling physically and mentally under the strain. She tearfully filled out the appropriate forms, but then a glance at the frail and pathetic-looking old man staring uncomprehendingly into a void moved her to tear the papers up and usher him out the door. She returned later in the day and the same scene was repeated. Only on the third visit that night was she able to accept the inevitable.

⌒

A stodgy middle-age matron who brought in her husband ran truer to form. The psychiatry intern who interviewed the couple had spent the entire day witnessing too many callous demonstrations of family relationships, and on this occasion permitted himself the luxury of sarcasm.

"And tell me, Mrs. Smith, what seems so wrong with your husband that you think he needs to go to a state hospital?"

"Oh, I dunno. He's just not as good as he was. He forgets things sometimes and he dribbles in his pants sometimes. . . . He's just not like he was."

"Tell me, Mrs. Smith, according to these forms you've filled out you have been married thirty-eight years, right?"

"Yeah."

"And your husband had a pretty good trade until he stopped working a couple of years ago?"

"Yeah, that's right."

"And he made a pretty good living most of the time?"

"Yeah."

"And he took pretty good care of you all those years; didn't mistreat you?"

"Oh no, he didn't mistreat me."

"And now you're telling me that after almost forty years of supporting you, he forgets things once in a while and sometimes wets his pants and you want to put him away in a state mental institution?"

"Yeah, that's right."

Next case.

5

The Iron Man

Growing Old Is One Thing; Doing It Gracefully Quite Another

MacPherson was rusting to death and there was nothing he could do to stop it. In a way, he thought it an appropriate fate for one whose bony and cartilaginous hinges had been so over-worked for so long. Yet he continued to resent the loss of his strength and mobility as he struggled against the inexorable freeze that continued to descend upon his bodily parts.

At eighty he was a far cry from the four-letter athlete of his high school days—track, baseball, football, and wrestling—but it was a sport far removed from the high school scene that was the source of his physical downfall. Midway through college, restless and without direction, he had decided upon a crack at the military life. He had joined the cavalry because, despite the practical disappearance of horses on the battlefield and their displacement by armored vehicles, a vestige of the old cavalry life remained. The unit he joined still maintained a stable of horses with which they could participate in equestrian events throughout the country. It was his fascination and growing af-fection for these magnificent beasts that led MacPherson to this decision, and soon he had added horsemanship to his other athletic accomplishments. Before long he was participating in jumping events, not only within the military establishment but also in competition with other teams composing the "horsey set" on the national and international scene.

An occasional fall from a mount is part and parcel of such sport, and Mac had his share. With his own desire for perfec-tion and an intense competitive spirit, perhaps he had more than his share of such mishaps as he pushed himself and his mounts to superlative performances. Eventually the accidents began to take a toll on the young man and, on one occasion, after landing on his lower back, he was confined to bed for more than a week. This episode seemed to open a door to inca-pacity, and with each subsequent fall the periods of enforced bed rest became longer and the ability to perform more limited.

So affected had his riding skills become through these accidents that, although he might be considered nearly normal in terms of civilian life, the military surgeons thought him no longer fit for service and he was discharged as physically disabled.

At the age of thirty, mustered out of the service, Dan Mac-Pherson was, in a real sense, a has-been at an age when most of his contemporaries were normally focused only on the future. Yet, despite his disappointment at having been eliminated from the sporting life he had chosen, his participation in all those national and international events had served him well. To those who closely followed such competitions, many of them rich and influential, Dan had become well known, not only for his riding and jumping expertise but also for his rugged good looks, his engaging personality, and a native intelligence unobscured by the fact that he lacked the academic credentials to prove it.

It was one of those enthusiasts, who also happened to be a major industrialist, who recognized MacPherson's potential and decided to take him under his wing. The same spirit of competition and desire to succeed on the track, the older man recognized, might serve to great advantage within the business world. He offered Dan a starting position in his firm and soon, in a very different sense, MacPherson was once again "off and running."

Thanks to his native ability and inexhaustible energy, Macpherson advanced rapidly upward through the echelons of the firm. And although he no longer could ride without fear of further damaging his back, MacPherson was able to participate in a number of more pedestrian sports within his capability: tennis, golf, etc. His climb up the corporate ladder was not, however, uninterrupted. Periodic physical disability continued to plague him. It was not often that a sporting event put him out of commission; oftentimes it was only the simple twisting of his back as he reached over for a paper or leaned over to pick up a small object from the floor. At any such time any slight unpredictable movement might result in his being bedridden and in traction for weeks. It was the threat of this that led to his curtailing any unnecessary sporting activity and a growing determination to seek a solution.

After more than ten years of repeated hospitalizations when his back "went out," he underwent sophisticated testing which revealed that it was a disc problem that was the cause of it all. A portion of one of these biological shock absorbers between two vertebrae in the lower back was protruding out of its normal position (herniating) and impinging on a nerve exiting from the spinal cord. Then as now, surgeons were not enthusiastic about attempting to correct such problems by operative intervention; the results are only fifty-fifty in terms of complete success. However, by the time MacPherson had found the surgeon who was reported to have "golden hands" in this regard, even this usually conservative practitioner needed little prodding. The reason was that, in addition to the recurrent attacks of lower back pain, often shooting down the left thigh, true weakness and muscle wasting had begun to appear in the affected limb.

Fortunately, the results of the surgery were spectacular. The back pain not only disappeared post-operatively but also the deterioration in function had been arrested, and thanks to a vigorous rehabilitation program that followed the surgery, strength and mobility were fully restored to the affected leg. Soon Dan was back again on the tennis and squash courts, out on the golf links, and indulging in all his athletic pursuits with the exception of horseback riding. Even he was not foolhardy enough to invite another round of disasters by risking this.

For nearly twenty years he continued to enjoy a satisfying professional and athletic life without a single mishap. Then one day, in attempting to rise up on his water skis at the lake on which the family summer vacation home was located, he found he could not maintain a grip on the tow bar with his left hand. The damned thing kept slipping out of his grasp. This was not a totally devastating experience, maybe just the effects of getting older, maybe a little arthritis in the hands, Dan thought. After all, he realized, he was no longer twenty-five and there were few men of his age that were still attempting to skim along the waves this way.

Giving up water skiing was no great sacrifice. He could still snow ski, jog, and play basketball and tennis, even succeeding once in a while in taking a set from his sons, who were then in their twenties.

A year or two after that failed attempt at water skiing, a new unusual symptom appeared. MacPherson began to have a distinct impression that the hairs on his left forearm were standing erect. Yet, when he closely compared them to those on the right forearm, there was no difference, both sides identically normal in appearance. The symptom actually had nothing to do with hair. It was a hypersensitivity of the sensory nerves supplying the skin of that forearm, one of nature's nasty little tricks: the development of supernormal sensitivity in an area supplied by a nerve that is about to give out and then result in total numbness and perhaps paralysis as it undergoes complete deterioration. It was a disc problem once again asserting itself. However, this time the disc was located much higher up, affecting the spinal cord in the region at the base of the neck. Now not only was the left leg to be disabled but the arm as well. Although this time around pain was not a prominent symptom, weakness and a lack of control of his left-sided extremities more than made up for it. Soon it was not discouragement about not being able to run around on a tennis court that was of concern to Mac-Pherson, but the fear that in the near future he might not even be able to walk without assistance.

The golden-handed surgeon had long since retired from

practice, but when importuned by Macpherson for a substitute, he referred his old patient to a new man whom he felt to be a worthy successor. Both men warned Macpherson that he had been very fortunate the first time around and that a guarantee of equally good results with a new operation could not be made. Nevertheless, there was no hesitation on the patient's part to proceed.

The results of the new surgical attempt to remove the new problematic disc in the upper spine were not so spectacular this time around. Although the surgeon was convinced that the rapid progression of weakness and wasting of the limbs was arrested post-operatively, subjectively, Dan could notice no improvement in his abilities and even suspected that the process was continuing to advance, albeit at a much slower rate. Within a few months, he came to the realization that not only would he never be able again to participate in any sports but also that even the mundane task of walking across a room would pose a significant problem for as far as he could see into the future. A southpaw from birth, he had to teach himself to write with the right hand when his left could no longer securely grasp a pen or pencil.

His wife and children joined his physician in urging him to seek some assistance, especially for his problems in ambulation. A brace might offer some support, or at least the use of a cane might avert a serious fall and hip fracture, head injury, or even brain damage. The proud, stubborn old man refused even in spite of the embarrassment he suffered when on several occasions his weaving along a street had prompted local observers to suspect someone in acute difficulty, a developing stroke, an insulin reaction, or even alcoholism. Upon viewing Dan's attempts at walking, anyone could easily have been led to believe this. His head swayed back and forth constantly as he struggled to maintain his center of gravity. Each time the left foot was raised from the ground it seemed to take on a life of its own;

this began with it inscribing an unpredictable arc of activity, swinging wildly about until it convulsively fell to earth once more, perhaps only a few inches ahead of its partner on the right.

With age, many of us mellow. We recognize that the decline of physical power is inevitable and are able to take comfort in the knowledge that this is the natural order of things. We learn to appreciate aspects of life that youth barely notices: the blooming of a flower, a sunset, the sounds of birds singing and the wind rustling through the trees, the smell and laughter of our grandchildren. We are glad simply to be alive. Dan MacPherson would have none of it. Every diminishment in physical capacity he looked upon as an affront to his existence. He resented each iota lost, not knowing quite whom to blame as he immersed himself in bitterness and frustration.

In a way this was admirable, not willingly giving up any ground, especially in view of the fact that his mental powers remained totally intact. Even after he retired from his long-held executive position, he was still sought out for advice and found it easy to set himself up as a successful consultant. He simply set up an office in his retirement home after moving from the metropolis. Thanks to computers, fax, e-mail, and the rest of modern business technology, he managed to function efficiently with the assistance of only a single secretary who arrived each day to sort the mail and messages.

MacPherson's great gift, thanks to his long and varied experience in business, was the ability to size up the worth of any company that some larger firm might be interested in acquiring. This required him to travel a good deal, something he actually enjoyed even though his family feared for his safety as he finished off his seventies and entered the ninth decade of life. It was only for distant travel that Mac relented and agreed to use a cane to help himself get about.

Embarking on a new venture was never a problem. Dan was

usually well rested before setting out, and the prospect of a "big deal" always seemed to invigorate him. It was the return trip that he dreaded. Having moved from a large city to his suburban home, he found that his cross-country trips always had to end with a flight from a major airport to his local field. Unlike the major terminals with their jetways that swing out and accordionlike connect to a plane's passenger exit after the craft has come to a halt and taxied up to the terminal, no such facilities were available at MacPherson's local airport. The aircraft simply parked out on the airstrip and an L-shaped stairway was rolled up to the exit to allow the passengers to descend. It was then a hike, all men and women for themselves, from the airstrip to the terminal.

With each home landing, MacPherson worried just how far he would have to walk this time to make it to the terminal. The airline personnel had long ago given up on the offer of a wheelchair; they knew how ornery their frequent passenger was in his refusal, even if they could not guess at his own insecurity with each landing.

On one occasion, after the plane had come to a halt and the seatbelt sign was turned off, MacPherson, as was his custom, waited until the cabin had been emptied of all the passengers within his view. "No need to hold anyone else up because I happen to be falling apart," he thought to himself. When the aisle seemed clear, MacPherson hauled himself to his feet, steadied himself with his cane grasped in his right hand, and then wobbled uncertainly down the aisle to the exit. Step by step he slowly descended the stair-ramp until he reached the bottom. Some distance ahead of him he observed the last of the other passengers scurrying across a seemingly endless expanse of concrete toward the terminal.

An uneasiness bordering on fear began to grip him as he calculated the odds for and against his own success at navigating this passage. While he hesitated, he heard a clunking sound behind him. He turned to see a small dark figure with a cane in his left hand descending slowly, one step at a time. The man who joined Dan at the foot of the stairs was even older and more feeble-looking than he. Nonetheless there was a certain flair about him with his full-length navy winter coat and a derby cocked to one side on his head.

There were a few days' growth of whiskers sprouting from his ruddy cheeks, Mac noted, as the old man's bright blue eyes peered past him in the direction of the terminal. Like Dan, he too was probably musing upon the prospect of this trek. Suddenly a smile lit up his face as he turned to Mac.

"Ya wanna race?"

At that moment as Dan gazed into the eyes of his new companion, a feeling of warmth, hardly familiar but not quite forgotten, began to envelop him. It was of humor, humility, understanding, and camaraderie in equal parts. With his own free hand he grasped the arm of the other.

"Let's go!"

And the two old men headed for home—as fast as their legs would carry them.

6

WASTE

WHAT'S LEFT OF A LIFE

Once a week the San Francisco Police Department made a practice of scouring under the bridges and around the shabby alleys of the Mission District for those among the city's derelicts who might be in need of medical attention. These searches usually took place on a Friday or Saturday night, and the police would deposit their complement of damaged humanity at the Emergency Room of the San Francisco General Hospital, where medical personnel would then take charge.

Once within the portals of the hospital, these unfortunate creatures would first be taken by gloved and gowned attendants to a special room that had been reserved for their reception. It was there that their clothes were removed for disinfection or burning and the patients, themselves, would be immersed in a tub containing various chemicals devised to destroy or at least seriously disable the collection of lice, ticks, "crabs," and occasional maggots that had nested with them.

After the delousing procedures, the patients would be draped in hospital gowns and placed in a holding ward for examination by the resident doctors. Almost all were acutely intoxicated but also suffered from long-term effects of chronic alcoholism and malnutrition: cirrhosis of the liver, peripheral and central nervous system disorders, dementia, tuberculosis, etc.

One evening as the latest group was laid out for inspection, the distinctive demeanor of one of these men caught the medical resident's eye. Propped up by two or three pillows bunched behind him, he was as dirty and wasted as the rest. Initially, the most striking feature about him were his legs, upon which the scabs and many sores had become confluent, giving them the appearance of two brown tree trunks protruding from beneath the hem of the hospital gown. As the doctor's gaze shifted to the head of the bed, past the patiently folded hands in the lap, he took note of the man's face—weather-beaten, unshaved, toothless, but with remarkable eyes that were brilliantly light blue, piercing and intelligent. In striking contrast to the dazed and blunted attitudes of his compatriots, this man seemed quite alert and observant. The medical resident found himself unable to resist fixing his eyes on the patient's own. After a few moments of this staring contest the patient smilingly inquired, "Are you gazing at me askance, young man?"

This was not the usual kind of repartee that the hospital staff were accustomed to hear from such patients, and later the doctor made some inquiries of some old hands who had worked in the emergency room for many years. He learned that in earlier times the man in question had been one of San Francisco's most prominent lawyers. He also enjoyed a statewide reputation and at one time had been retained by officials in Sacramento as the primary legal architect in a redrafting of the California State Constitution. And then he took to drink. "Askance," indeed.

7

MARKING TIME AT HILLCREST HOME

HOW ONE YOUNG DOCTOR ATTEMPTED
TO BEAT THE SYSTEM—AND FAILED

Dr. Lorenzo Garibaldi had a problem: his next assignment was to be at Hillcrest Home.

As part of the three-year training program in Internal Medicine at his teaching hospital, each member of the house staff was plucked from the turmoil of the acute care services and deposited for a six-week tour of duty at Hillcrest, a county-owned facility for the aged, infirm, and the simply socially inadequate with no other place to go.

According to the brochure distributed to new members of the house staff training program, the Hillcrest Home experience provided "a valuable exposure to the medical problems of the aged and an opportunity to learn the value and application of supportive medical care for the geriatric population." In actual practice, to the doctors assigned to Hillcrest it really meant a leisurely hiatus inserted in their otherwise hectic schedules. One could enjoy forty-two straight nights of uninterrupted sleep.

Most of the medical residents looked forward to Hillcrest. It could provide an opportunity for catching up on one's medical reading. But one seldom did. In the winter months one was more likely to catch up on one's television viewing, and in spring and summer the major redeeming feature of the place, its spacious lawns and shade trees, offered hours of peaceful repose. One drawback to the assignment was the requirement for twenty-four-hour daily attendance on the premises with the exception of Sundays. This precluded the usual off-duty occupations of the house staff: earning additional funds to supplement their meager salaries by "moonlighting" at understaffed local hospitals and the general dissipation of such ill-gotten gains in various evening pursuits. Thus, like it or not, it was a period for physical and mental unwinding.

This would not do for Lorenzo Garibaldi. This brash and energetic second-year resident was neither of the magnificent Medici line nor a blood relation to the unifier of Italy, but all his life, it seemed, he had been intent on living up to his prepossessing name. He had been first in his medical school class, but there, as well as in his postgraduate training, he was content not only to excel but also to do so with a flair that invariably managed to diminish the stature of his mentors.

His specialty involved his discovering a patient with a previously unrecognized rare disease and then confronting his superiors with his "suspicions" (already secretly proved by objective laboratory evidence). Following the professorial pooh-poohs that would more often than not follow, Lorenzo would then prove himself right and them wrong with a presentation of the completed workup. The pooh-poohs were becoming much less frequent as Lorenzo continued to haunt the hospital medical wards.

A brilliant firebrand like Garibaldi was totally unsuited for Hillcrest Home. He did not need to catch up on the medical literature; he was always right up to date. He hated television. He was incapable of relaxing. Lorenzo, who thoroughly enjoyed his spoiled-brat medical reputation, despaired of the boredom that threatened to engulf him at Hillcrest, although the medical staff that supervised as well as suffered him at the hospital had mixed feelings about his imminent departure. He certainly was stimulating to have around the hospital, but then, no one liked the feeling of being a deflated balloon.

As the departure date approached, Lorenzo pondered his future moves at Hillcrest. Was there any table there to be overturned? Where could he thrust the next needle into a puffed-up officialdom? The likelihood of his turning up any rare diseases was exceedingly small among the nearly one thousand mostly elderly men and women who would be under his care. The turnover was nothing like that at the city hospital clinics, where he had been able to discover an occasional "ringer" to baffle the hospital attending staff. Furthermore, even if he did come upon something potentially remarkable, he would not be able to prove his diagnosis at Hillcrest. There were insufficient laboratory facilities available to work up any patient on the premises. Medical care at the home consisted of shipping any patient with an acute illness off to the city hospital.

It was the basic inadequacy of medical care at Hillcrest that gave Garibaldi the plan for his newest escapade. The blurb in the hospital bulletin notwithstanding, quality of care was not where it could or should have been. Except for the presence of a house officer on site and the shuttle to the city hospital when necessary, attention to the medical needs of the inmates was practically nonexistent. Well, not while Garibaldi was around. What better way to tweak the proverbial whiskers of the administration than by taking its written pronouncements literally and actually providing proper medical surveillance for all the patients assigned to him? He would place an official up-to-date medical progress note on the chart of every patient in the institution, a feat that had never been attempted in the entire history of Hillcrest Home.

To begin with, was this possible? Garibaldi checked the mathematics of the situation. There were exactly 987 patients confined to the institution at this time. He could not do a formal interview and physical examination on all. The former alone, what with language difficulties and frequent mentation problems among the inmates, would unconscionably prolong the process. But if he dispensed with medical history–taking and simply relied on a five-minute review of the previous notes, followed by a quick physical examination covering all the major organ systems, he might well complete a reasonably reliable examination in twenty minutes.

With four hours of clinic in the morning, three in the afternoon, and two every evening, he could complete 27 examinations each working day, 162 in each six-day working week, and 972 within the six-week period. Throw in a few extra hours on a couple of Sundays and he could make up the balance to reach

987 by the end of his rotation. And then, triumphantly, he would hand in his report to the unsuspecting chief of medicine upon his return to the hospital.

The Sunday evening he arrived at Hillcrest, he deposited his bags in the medical resident quarters and immediately proceeded to the Patient Record Room, where he withdrew the files of the subjects for the first week's examinations. The nursing staff were a little surprised at the energetic beginnings of the new doctor, but had no doubt that he would come to his senses within a week or two.

By the end of the first week, Lorenzo knew he would be able to finish the task he had set for himself. He had allotted more than enough time for his brief but businesslike patient evaluations. He had seen 171 patients, 9 more than the minimum scheduled according to his plan.

Two weeks passed, and he was still ahead of schedule. There were some patients with relatively minor chronic medical problems, but orders for medications were dutifully renewed and the drugs administered. That second Saturday night he crossed off patient number 336.

During the second two weeks he sent three patients to the city hospital: one with pneumonia, one with a possible coronary attack, and the third with possible appendicitis. It was 652 down and 335 to go.

After a month of performing these examinations, Garibaldi developed the ability to predict almost with a glance at each patient the content of the note he would ultimately assign to him. As they entered the office, he would immediately categorize them: "chronic brain syndrome," "emphysema," "old cerebrovascular accident (CVA)," "senility and debility," . . . He could almost have devised a set of rubber stamps, one for each category, with blanks left only for the name, age, and hospital number of the patient.

As the first flush of satisfaction passed after he realized the potential success of his undertaking, his efforts became mechanical, then boring, and finally, toward the end, deadeningly monotonous. The parade of humanity that shuffled in and out of the little examining room became a blur.

As the purpose of his efforts continued to diminish in importance to him, the awareness of larger issues grew in Garibaldi's mind. The patients no longer seemed like pawns to be played with in his latest challenge to authority. They were, rather, victims of a mindless and heartless bureaucracy, compartmentalized out of the mainstream of society—as was he, Garibaldi, for these six weeks of his life.

At the beginning of the sixth week Dr. Lorenzo Garibaldi finally came of age. His first patient that Monday morning was in his late seventies and, having been at Hillcrest since the age of twenty-four, he was one of the inmates who had been in the facility the longest. As a youth he might have been characterized as "inadequate personality" or perhaps "simple schizophrenic." He had no complaints.

Lorenzo began listlessly to leaf through the hospital chart presented him. He came to a page dated "June 2, 1935" and read, "No further evidence of upper respiratory infection. Appears well." The next entry began "March 19, 1946. Called to see patient . . ." It had taken almost eleven years for someone to take notice again.

Garibaldi looked at the patient sitting impassively before him. He then looked out the window, and for the first time took notice of the lush green laws beckoning in the early morning sunlight. Before dismissing the patient and leaving the room himself, he entered his final brief note on a Hillcrest patient's hospital chart: "Status unchanged."

8

The Case of the Baffling Boy: Chapter One

An Early Lesson in Child Abuse

Dr. Kaufman was puzzled by the records concerning Richard, the five-year-old boy whom he had agreed to evaluate. The adult nephrologist who had seen the child a month before felt that someone like Kaufman, a pediatrician who specialized in kidney disorders, might better be able to get to the bottom of the case than he. Kaufman was fortunate in at least one respect: as with all childhood diseases, the history of the case was not a particularly long one.

About a year earlier, the child's mother, a nurse, had noticed he was passing rusty-colored urine, suspected bleeding (hematuria), and brought him to a urologist in the distant city in which they had then been living. At that time the surgeon felt that dilatation of the urethra, the tubular structure running from the bladder through the penis, was in order, and this apparently solved the problem temporarily. After an asymptomatic period of about ten or twelve months, with the family now settled in Kaufman's area, the mother again reported the darkening of the urine, but now, in addition to this, noted recurring fevers in the boy, with temperatures spiking as high as 103 degrees Fahrenheit at times.

Kaufman was determined to evaluate the case thoroughly and had the child hospitalized so that he could be observed carefully. The mother cooperated fully and was at the child's bedside almost constantly, assisting the hospital staff in charting temperatures and obtaining various urine specimens for analysis. Of all the urine samples obtained among the many that tested positive by Hemastick for blood, only two samples actually showed red blood cells on microscopic examination.

What puzzled Kaufman the most was the intermittency of the problem and the relative paucity of other significant findings relating either to the kidney or the blood. All X-ray studies, including the intravenous pyelogram to outline the kidneys and their drainage, had been normal. On several occasions, he had taken Richard's temperature himself and found it normal. He had also intensively scanned slides of fresh urinary sediment (an aliquot obtained after centrifugation to concentrate formed urine elements) and except for those two odd samples, found no red cells or other substances that could account for the positive laboratory tests for blood that were so frequent.

The presence of red cells themselves was not completely essential to the diagnosis of hematuria. The red cell walls could have dissolved in the urine, and free hemoglobin in the urine could have accounted for the positive tests. Alternatively, red cells could have been breaking down in the patient's blood stream before reaching the kidney and causing the positive testing of the urine. But no evidence of this was forthcoming. Urine samples sent to specialized laboratories revealed no trace of hemoglobin determined by other, more refined methods of analysis despite the positive Hemastick tests that continued to confound him.

Because of the frequently high fevers, an infection was suspected. But the urinary sediment showed no pus cells, the presence of which would usually be an indication of such a disorder. The cultures of the urine for bacteria were even stranger than those tests for red cell pigment. All showed no growth except those two samples that actually contained red cells on microscopic examination. It was in these that two highly respected microbiologists returned reports of a growth of organisms that they were amazed to find as a possible cause of a urinary tract infection in a five-year-old boy: the typical flora found in the adult vagina.

Such infections had nonetheless been reported as rarities and were extremely difficult to treat. If this was indeed the cause of the fevers, then postponing antibiotic therapy might put the kidneys at some risk of tissue destruction as a result of the untreated infection. Therefore a course of antibiotic therapy was attempted to see if this would have any effect on the fevers. The antibiotic chosen was one that was felt to be effective yet relatively free of side effects. Soon after the therapy was begun, Richard began having attacks of severe vomiting. Although this particular toxic effect was considered especially unusual for the drug being used, they decided to discontinue it nonetheless. The boy and his mother were sent home temporarily while Kaufman and his associates awaited the results of additional laboratory data that was pending.

At this point they had begun to consider the possibility that the pigment discoloring the urine was not from the blood at all but actually myoglobin, the pigment that is one of the components of muscle. The child might be a victim of some type of muscle-wasting disease and the red cell theory a "red herring" after all. The mother was informed of this and told to return with Richard in several days to resume evaluation with special attention now focusing on the muscular system.

She arrived at the hospital with Richard cradled in her arms. He could not walk, she claimed, and demanded that the nephrologist take samples (biopsies) of both kidneys and various muscles to determine the source of the urinary pigment. There was yet another surprise in store for Kaufman and his colleagues, for the tests for myoglobin in the urine had likewise proved negative as were the tests of Richard's muscular function and metabolism about to prove. Furthermore, as the boy later protested that he could not move from the hospital bed to the adjoining bathroom without assistance, the mention of a large needle as a stimulus to the desired action resulted in his immediate "recovery," with him bolting immediately from the bed to the other side of the room.

By this time the physicians' suspicions, perhaps in retrospect a little belatedly, were fully aroused. Why was it that all the urine specimens that Kaufman had obtained personally were always normal but those obtained throughout the day through the "good offices" of Richard's mother so frequently tainted? Why, in spite of all the fever spikes, could Kaufman never personally record one nor could he recall placing his hands on Richard's body and sensing it to be clearly febrile to his touch? Why the maternal overreaction to the possibility of muscle disease? What was the meaning of an episode that one of the nurses reported soon after the antibiotic therapeutic trial had begun? On that occasion, when she had entered the boy's room she had found the mother standing over her son with the pills saying very definitely, "You are going to take these pills now Richie, but you *know* you are going to vomit them up, don't you? Vomit them right up!"

The next part of the investigation was more in the realm of Baker Street ratiocination than renal disease. The doctors obtained the use of an unusual kind of playroom on the pediatric service. It contained a special one-way mirror so that patterns of child play could be observed by psychiatrists and psychologists from an adjoining room while the toddlers were aware of nothing more than an ordinary-appearing mirror on the wall. Richard and his mother were brought to this room one morning under the pretext that a new visiting kidney specialist would be meeting them to evaluate the case. Kaufman and his associates left the room, ostensibly to fetch the new consultant, leaving the two alone. While they were gone, they instructed the mother, she was to measure the boy's temperature and secure a fresh sample of urine for inspection.

Her first act, following the doctors' exit, was to survey the room critically and then approach the mirror through which she was being observed. She cupped both hands over her brows and pressed them against the glass in an attempt to peer through at the very doctors that were observing her. As she attempted this, two doctors immediately outside the playroom were cued to begin speaking in loud voices about the renal problems of the young boy they were treating. The sound of their voices penetrating partially through the closed door reassured the woman, and she set about her business.

First she went to the sink in the corner of the room and placed the thermometer under the hot water tap for a few minutes. Checking the reading and finding it too high for her purposes, she carefully shook it down to a level of between 102 and 103 degrees. She then had Richard void into an empty container that had been provided, half filling it. Following this, she opened her purse from which she withdrew a jar containing some dark-colored fluid and added a portion of it to the fresh urine specimen of her son's and seated herself to await the return of the physicians.

Kaufman reentered the room and, in as even a manner as he could manage, informed the woman that he and his colleagues had observed through the special mirror everything that she had done in their presumed absence from the room. She simply chose to ignore the matter of the thermometer and addressed the charge of her having tampered with the urine.

"What could I have possibly put in that urine to make it look bloody?"

Kaufman's extensive recent reading on the subject of urine testing by various commercial stick devices had not been in vain. "You could have simply added any iodine-containing compound to the urine. This will give a positive test for blood on the stick test and explains why we never found any blood when we analyzed the urine specifically for that by chemical analysis." He did pursue the source of the truly positive blood samples and the type of bacteriologic growth they provided but the woman's menstrual flow could have provided a logical explanation.

The mother stormed out with her son intact—or at least his kidneys and muscles unviolated by any surgical assaults upon them.

The next step in the process was almost as difficult as those preceding it. The father, a rough-hewn cross-country truck operator/owner who was seldom home, had to be informed of the results of the doctors' investigations. When he finally appeared to discuss "a matter of some urgency regarding your son," his fierce appearance did not make broaching the subject of his wife's odd tendencies any easier for a mild-mannered and diminutive pediatrician.

"Mr. J_____, we know how concerned you must have been about Richard. And your wife, with her nursing background, must have kept you informed about what we . . ."

"Nursing background? She's no nurse. The most she ever did in a hospital was work as a volunteer for a year or two when we lived in Ohio."

"Well then, this sort of fits in with what I have to tell you."

The father remained impassive throughout the entire recounting of the complicated story. He sighed, "I'm not surprised," and then went on to inform Kaufman of an older child about whom the pediatrician had been told relatively little. The child had had many emotional complaints, finally leading to a year's treatment by a child psychiatrist. At the end of the treatment period, the psychiatrist had reported to the father that basically there was nothing wrong with the child; he was essentially normal. The mother, however, the psychiatrist felt, was quite ill and much in need of psychiatric help. The mother refused, and the father acquiesced in this decision.

Richard's problem and that of his brother occurred some years ago, long before the medical profession, the courts, and society in general had caught up with the problems of child abuse.* Nothing was ever done along these lines, and neither Richard's ultimate fate nor that of his mother was ever determined by Kaufman or any of the others who had worked along with him on the case of the baffling boy.

* Some years later, as pediatricians and psychiatrists uncovered a number of cases similar to that described here, they were categorized as a specific type of child abuse. See Roy Meadow, "Munchausen Syndrome by Proxy." *Arch Dis Childhood* 57 (1982): 92–98.

9

EDDY

A PATIENT FOCUSED ON SELF-DESTRUCTION
ELUDES HIS DOCTOR'S CARE

We tend to think of patients' attitudes and willpower in terms of either the tenacity with which some cling to life or else the ease with which others relinquish their hold upon it. What was remarkable about Eddy was his unrelenting determination after a period of years to escape it until he finally met with success.

He first came to our attention when, at the age of fourteen, he was referred to our cardiology unit for evaluation of a heart murmur. On the basis of our examination we concluded that he had rheumatic heart disease, with minor leaks of both the aortic and mitral valves. Since the heart chambers were still not enlarged and the patient asymptomatic, no therapy was indicated other than the administration of penicillin to prevent recurring attacks of rheumatic fever, which might result in further damage to the heart valves. The penicillin could be taken orally with a supply given to the patient on discharge from the hospital, or else the patient could return monthly for a single injection of a long-acting form. We preferred the latter option since it gave us a better chance at following such patients closely and ensuring that the medication was actually taken as prescribed. Eddy, however, insisted on the oral route and was lost to our follow-up for a period of three years. Whether he ever took his medication at home was questionable. Antibiotic prophylaxis against heart valve infection (endocarditis) with dental procedures, etc., was also advised but probably not undertaken.

Our next meeting occurred in the emergency room of the city hospital where Eddy, now seventeen, had been admitted with severe coughing and shortness of breath. His lungs were congested (pulmonary edema). The left ventricle of his heart, overloaded by the chronic leak of the mitral valve separating it from the upper chamber (atrium) had finally failed and, as a result of this, blood was backing up in his lungs. Emergency medical measures brought the immediate situation under control, and Eddy was admitted to the Cardiac Care Unit, where several days later he was able to undergo cardiac catheterization to better evaluate the severity of both leaking valves on the left side of his heart and determine whether or not both the aortic and mitral valves would need replacement. The aortic valve was found to be leaking only moderately, but the cineangiogram of the mitral valve showed that it was almost completely incapable of closing adequately due to the scarring and shrinkage caused by the probable repeated attacks of rheumatic fever and the constant wear and tear of daily living. It would have to be replaced by an artificial mechanical valve.

The surgery went smoothly, and the hemodynamic result after insertion of the prosthetic valve was gratifying. However, a major problem with mechanical valve replacements is that their surfaces often serve as foci upon which blood clots (thrombi) tend to form. These thrombi may interfere with the proper opening and closing of the valve; they may also prove a threat to the patient by their propensity to break off and be carried to vital organs such as the brain, kidney, or the heart itself through the coronary arteries (thromboembolism). For this reason, cardiologists will use drugs to reduce the coagulability of the blood in such patients post-operatively. Such drugs may be administered for several months, years, or even indefinitely, depending upon the characteristics of the valve inserted. Thus Eddy was duly anticoagulated prior to his discharge from the hospital and instructed to return periodically for reevaluations of his cardiac status and the adequacy of his blood-clotting control. As with all such patients, he was advised to avoid traumatizing himself in any way in view of the risk of excessive hemorrhage following such events due to the anticoagulant medication.

In less than two months following discharge from the hospital, Eddy was returned to us with a painfully swollen and discolored ankle. He and some friends had been roof hopping. Eddy had stumbled, twisting the ankle joint into which and around which a considerable amount of blood had accumulated.

The bleeding was controlled with antidotes to the anticoagulant and local measures. This initial warning sign of his tendency toward self-destruction was passed off as youthful high jinks and, following resumption of his anticoagulation drug, he was discharged from the hospital with warnings to take better care of himself. More substantial proof of his intent to the contrary soon followed.

Eddy, a handsome, blond Hollywood juvenile type, began his practice of attending dances at which he would flirt with the girlfriends of the biggest and toughest-looking young men there. These imbroglios often resulted in a pummeling that put him back in the hospital with multiple hemorrhagic bruises. When the ploy of baiting other youngsters was not found to work with sufficient regularity, Eddy took to various forms of rowdyism that invariably brought him to the attention of the police. He never went peacefully to the station and thereby incurred repeated beatings from the police officers, who were unaware of his medical condition. It soon became apparent that the risk of his bleeding to death as a result of his frequent escapades was probably a greater threat to his survival than that of thrombus formation on the valve. His anticoagulation treatment was discontinued.

Fortunately, Eddy did not prove to be prone to clot formation, and for the remaining years of his life did not suffer any episodes of thromboembolism. However, following the cessation of the anticoagulants, Eddy's antisocial behavior took a different form as he began to ingest and later deal in a variety of stimulant and depressive drugs, mostly amphetamines and barbiturates. When the police finally caught up with him and he went on trial, the court requested a medical evaluation. In our opinion, Eddy had amply demonstrated that he was more in need of psychiatric help than incarceration. Because of his youthful good looks, we were especially concerned about the possibility of homosexual rape in prison resulting in physical harm as well as adding to his mental problems. Nonetheless, the penal route was the one selected by the court, and he spent the next three years in various prison facilities throughout the state.

When he was finally released, he had barely reached his twenty-third birthday. On a visit to us for an evaluation he was full of brave talk about the future, although it was now evident that he had begun to inject drugs under his skin and intravenously. Within six months he acquired an uncontrollable infection throughout his bloodstream as a result of an infection on his heart valve (bacterial endocarditis) and was admitted moribund to a local hospital where he died soon after.

We have often discussed the irony of his case: the completely satisfactory surgical result despite his complete lack of cooperation, and the ultimate negation of whatever we had achieved medically by his disturbed psyche. We wondered, but some contributing factors were all too apparent. In all the years we had treated him, we had never been able to reach his father. We spoke only once to his mother, who came to the hospital only late at night to sign the necessary consent forms for various procedures and not really to communicate with the doctors—or, apparently, even her son.

10

SMART ASS

A SLIP OF THE TONGUE

To some, mention of Chillingsworth will evoke memories of that sinister character in Hawthorne's tale of Puritan bigotry and spiritual survival, *The Scarlet Letter*. For me, the name has another connotation. It was what an aging eccentric chose to call his restaurant on Cape Cod some years ago. Each year, as we planned our two weeks of summer vacation in the sea and sand with our small children, we also looked forward to splurging for at least one night at that elegant establishment. The restaurant was done in the style of pre-revolutionary eighteenth-century France and, to match the décor, the waiters and waitresses were costumed in white linen and yellow satin. The ambience was matched only by the fine cuisine.

This year, as was our custom, as soon as we arrived on the Cape at our rented cottage, we called for reservations and arranged for a babysitter. We were to be joined by a medical school classmate and his wife who had just purchased a small home in Brewster. The day of our scheduled dinner, my friend called to ask if we would mind being joined by another physician and his wife, with whom my friends had become acquainted over the previous year and who were also visiting the Cape. A call to the restaurant indicated that there would be no problem accommodating six instead of four diners.

My wife and I were already seated at the time the four other guests arrived. I was in my early forties at the time and noticed that the newcomers were about twenty years older than my classmate and I. The husband was tall, well built, and athletic-looking with a rim of gray around a reddish pate. His wife was tiny, had obviously been quite pretty in her youth, and retained many traces of it.

The evening progressed famously, as the saying goes, with great food and drink encouraging our camaraderie. The new couple were charming, the husband expansive and amusing, the wife sweet, perhaps a little tentative, but nonetheless responsive to the good cheer with which she was surrounded. As always with doctors, the talk finally turned to the profession and, in the jocular spirit of the occasion, I thought I would pose a little puzzle to my two colleagues.

"What," I asked, "do you think the most accurate X-ray examination is?"

It was a trick question, of course, one I had gleaned from a recent article that I hoped the others had missed. The correct answer was X-rays of the skull. This was not because skull films were inherently simpler to interpret than other radiological examinations; in fact they could be very difficult to assess at times. The reason for the high batting average for radiologists with skull films was that the overwhelming majority of them would turn out to be normal. Fear of malpractice litigation had so intimidated emergency room physicians that whenever anyone walked in and even mentioned a bump on the head, a series of skull films would automatically be taken. Since so many unnecessary studies were being ordered on normal patients, it was the statistics of the situation that gave rise to such accuracy.

The two men pondered the question a few moments, suspecting some kind of catch, and hesitated to commit themselves. Observing their indecision, I could not contain myself.

"Skull films, of course," I exploded, and then began going into the detailed explanation of these results.

As I continued on, enveloped by my own enthusiasm, I failed to notice either the pained look on the faces of my friend and his wife or the deathly silence and withdrawal that had overtaken the other couple. Soon after this we parted ways. The evening, which had started off so well, had somehow ended on an inexplicably sad and deflated note.

The reason for this I learned from my classmate, who telephoned us the following morning. He told me about the other couple's seventeen-year-old son who, a year or two earlier, had returned home after a rather rambunctious party. Already tall and rugged like his father, in the flush of youth he was also prone to put it to the test and often became involved in adolescent rough-housing at such affairs. This was no exception, and as he entered the house his parents noticed his clothes in disarray and a bruise on his forehead.

"Maybe you should take him to the hospital for an X-ray?" the mother had suggested to her husband. This seemed a bit excessive to the father. When he questioned his son, he learned that there had been no loss of consciousness after his head had struck the floor at the party. He had no neurological evidence of any brain injury. All he complained of was a slight headache.

"Just let me get a good night's sleep and I'll be fine in the morning."

The mother again urged a trip to the hospital emergency room but was overruled by her husband and son.

The hours of the next morning wore on without the appearance of their son at the breakfast table. Finally, a visit to his bedroom provided the reason. The autopsy demonstrated a small skull fracture. One of the bone fragments had turned inward, severing a tiny artery. During the night the small but constant pumping of blood into the rigid cranium had compressed the brain with a large blood clot, leading to the death of the young man.

Some puzzle!

11

Victims All

Where to Draw the Line Where the
Doctor's Responsibility for the Patient
Leaves Off and the Patient's Determination
of His or Her Own Fate Begins?

One in nine American women are destined to develop breast cancer at some time during their lives, and Vera Cummings was convinced that she would be numbered among them.

This morbid obsession arose as a result of her grandmother's death from the disease. It did not help to know that an increased likelihood of developing breast cancer had been demonstrated only for first-degree relatives (daughters, sisters) and that having an affected grandmother or aunt, for example, had not been shown to be a risk factor for any individual. Neither this nor the knowledge that her own mother had lived well into her eighties without developing the disease provided any comfort. The threat of inevitability continued to hang over her, irrational but nonetheless real.

Perhaps it was such thoughts about her vulnerability that directed Vera to the study of medicine in the first place, although this might be stretching it too far. But after graduating from medical school and entering the specialty of radiology, Vera's drift into the field of mammography most certainly was not simply due to chance.

As for her personal style in the way she practiced her profession, she in no way resembled the feminist man-eaters often found upon the scene today. Vera was a child of the fifties and sixties when "ladylike" was not a dirty word and, despite the furor of feminism that followed, she always attempted to conform to this earlier model. This softness around the edges actually endeared her to her patients. Entering her fifties, Vera could easily assume the role of friend and confidante to the increasing number of older women coming to her after the frightening discovery of a lump in the breast. To the younger women who sought her out she could just as easily adopt the role of older sister or aunt.

Such mannerisms, however, did not serve her well in the macho male world of medicine, where, despite all her qualifications and certifications in radiology and its subspecialty components, she was often undervalued. Her desire to be absolutely confident in making a precise diagnosis in cases that were not clear-cut only made her seem tentative to her partners. Her painstaking approach to her work was considered simply too slow. The kind of solicitude that she invariably demonstrated to her patients was looked upon as unprofessional. No doubt such denigration, no matter how subtle, helped feed her fears that one day she might miss a lesion; she might unwittingly contribute to a late diagnosis; she might even be partly responsible, thereby, for additional pain and suffering or even the death of another woman. There then came that autumn afternoon when the sheriff's deputy entered her office with a summons, and she realized that her worst nightmare was about to become a reality.

It all began in a rather routine manner when, four years earlier, Mary Parker had appeared in the office, referred by Dr. James Bush, the obstetrician-gynecologist who had cared for her throughout her adulthood and who had delivered her two little girls, then three and five years of age. At the time this first mammogram was to be taken, Mary was only thirty-two.

Mary had complained earlier that day, on the morning she visited Bush, that for some weeks she had been feeling a lump in her left breast. She was particularly concerned about this because an aunt had recently died from breast cancer. The gynecologist could feel nothing out of the ordinary but, in order to reassure his patient, for whom he had developed a special affection over the years, he inserted a needle into the area she indicated and attempted to aspirate any material, normal or otherwise, that might be there. Only a few drops of fluid were obtained, and on microscopic examination the cellular elements all appeared normal.

To further reassure his patient and convince himself that he had not missed anything, he had sent Mary to Vera's office, requesting that Vera examine the breasts herself in conjunction with the X-ray study of the breasts, mammography. Vera had palpated the breasts carefully and could detect no unusual masses. The breasts were, however, firm and somewhat irregular or "lumpy" in the terminology generally used in such cases. This was certainly not unusual for a woman Mary's age, but it was nonetheless problematic from a strictly technical diagnostic viewpoint. Although breast cancer was rare in young women, with only one in two hundred cases of diagnosed breast cancer found in women between the ages of twenty and forty, it was among these women that physical examination and especially mammography, ordinarily an excellent diagnostic tool, tended to be less than satisfactory.

The problem is that young women in the child-bearing ages tend to have firm, dense breasts, frequently nodular or lumpy in consistency, making it difficult to distinguish by touch any abnormal masses from the normal breast tissue. Furthermore, during various phases of the menstrual cycle areas within the breast will often swell, sometimes painfully, and then subside. It is this same high density of the young female breast that makes it more difficult to use mammography to distinguish an abnormal mass, possibly a cancerous growth, from the surrounding normal tissue. A small neoplasm, especially, nestled within the dense tissue of a young woman's breast might be very difficult to detect, whereas the same neoplasm would be easy to demonstrate in older women in whom much of the normal breast tissue has been converted to fat, providing a clear background surrounding such abnormal growth.

In Mary's case no tumor could be seen on the mammogram. In the region Jim Bush had attempted to aspirate there was an irregular haziness a few inches in diameter that Vera thought might be related to that procedure. However, this turned up only in one view. When attempts were made to define it better with views of the breast taken at other angles, there was nothing at all to see. Vera rightfully concluded that it was probably an artifact of technique on the single view in which it appeared.

Following her review of the mammograms, Vera had gone out to the waiting room to reassure the patient. She had told Mary that many women in their childbearing years have recurrent swelling with regression in their breasts during their monthly cycle. She had advised Mary to avoid caffeine-containing beverages as well as chocolate, which contains another related substance that also tends to aggravate this condition. Vera knew that with such simple steps two-thirds of women with this complaint would have significant relief.

Given the age of the patient, the negative physical findings by two experienced physicians, and the negative mammogram, neither Vera nor Jim Bush felt it necessary to schedule a repeat mammogram as a follow up. Both were sure they told the patient—as all physicians do—that if the condition worsened or any new developments arose she could return to Dr. Bush's office. Vera also indicated to Mary that, although the chances of her having breast cancer were exceedingly small, no test was 100 percent accurate and at the bottom of the report was included the statement that "A negative X-ray report should not delay biopsy if a dominant or clinically suspicious mass is present since 4 to 8 percent of cancers are not identified by X-rays."

Vera's next meeting with Mary Parker took place about four months later. A telephone call had come from Jim Bush. In a tone that revealed some concern, he asked to bring Mary over to the radiology office personally for a repeat mammogram. She had suddenly appeared in his office with a golf ball–sized warm and tender mass in her left breast. A small amount of bloody material was oozing from the nipple. The bleeding had begun the day before when one of her daughters had accidentally bumped against her chest.

The mammography technician positioned the breast on the

small supporting platform of the X-ray device and lowered the screen to compress the tissues for better delineation of the structures within. With this maneuver, several ounces of bloody discharge were propelled explosively from the breast, covering parts of the machine, the floor, and the technician. The startled technician immediately reported this to Vera, who verified what had happened.

The first question that occurred to Vera was, "How could Mary, an intelligent young woman who incidentally worked in a hospital environment as a laboratory technician, sit idly by while this mass enlarged at such a terrifyingly rapid rate?" The testimony later given by Mary revealed the reason for the delay. Having been assured at that first visit by two physicians that she had nothing to worry about, she simply refused to recognize the significance of any new potentially ominous developments no matter how dramatic and rapidly occurring they were. Denial can be a very powerful emotion and a treacherous source of false comfort to a patient. Only when the bleeding began did the self-delusional bubble burst, forcing Mary to confront her illness.

Given her state of mind, it was only natural that Mary had convinced herself that she was told to return only if bleeding from the breast had occurred. Vera realized that for her own peace of mind Mary was compelled to believe this, despite the facts to the contrary. Yet, even following that disturbingly bloody event in the X-ray suite, Vera and Bush had good reason to believe that something other than cancer had accounted for it.

Bleeding from the breast is rare in breast cancer, occurring in fewer than 1 percent of patients as a presenting complaint, painless breast masses being overwhelmingly the norm. And when women do bleed from the breast, it is almost always the older women that have cancer as the cause; a variety of benign conditions usually account for this very troubling symptom in the vast majority of younger women. Vera, in nearly twenty years of practice and thousands upon thousands of patients examined, had seen women with this complaint only two or three times a year and these were always older women, usually well over fifty, with breast cancer. She had yet to observe this in any woman as young as Mary.

Following the demonstration of a sizable mass both on physical examination and mammography, it was decided to perform an ultrasound examination of the breast. This technique, although decidedly inferior to mammography in detecting suspected masses, is useful in determining whether an established mass is solid or filled with fluid. Benign, noncancerous conditions, such as cysts, are fluid-filled, while cancers are solid unless some breakdown of tissue within them has occurred as a result of the neoplasm outgrowing its blood supply, for example, or the neoplasm eroding a blood vessel in its vicinity.

Infections can also result in fluid-filled masses, collections of pus, and Mary's breast was certainly infected as cultures of the material obtained from her breast were to prove. A general surgeon was called in to manage the problem, and at the time he opened up the breast to allow drainage, he biopsied tissue in and around the mass for microscopic analysis. The pathologist indicated that the underlying cause of her complaint was indeed a cancer, a rapidly growing one, as indicated from the appearance of the cells that had been provided him.

Following the resolution of the superimposed infection, a modified radical mastectomy (removal of the entire breast and adjacent nodes but not the underlying chest muscles) was performed. One of the axillary lymph nodes obtained, two and a half centimeters in length (about an inch), upon sectioning, was shown to have had its contents completely replaced by cancer cells.

Because of the extent of the cancer beyond the borders of the breast, chemotherapy was clearly indicated, and this was administered over the next seven or eight months. Three years following the final weekly infusion of anti-cancer drugs, about four years since Mary had initially appeared in Vera's office, it became evident that the chemotherapy had not worked. Mary began to complain of chest pain, and X-rays of this area revealed that the cancer had metastasized to the lung. At this point a second course of chemotherapy was considered and even the possibility of a dramatic new and experimental treatment for breast cancer, bone marrow transplantation, was mentioned by the cancer specialist (oncologist) in charge of her case.

It was also at this time that Mary decided to consult a lawyer.

The validity of a case of medical malpractice depends upon two major premises: first, that the practitioner, either in terms of diagnosis or treatment, deviated from accepted standards of medical practice at the time; second, that such deviations resulted in compensable harm to the patient. The lawyers representing Mary Parker contended that both Jim Bush and Vera Cummings should be been held accountable for failure on both counts.

Regarding the first, at the trial it was the gynecologist who bore the brunt of the attack on his professionalism. Why had he ignored the complaint of his patient? Why had he not followed her more closely? Why had he allowed her to go undiagnosed and untreated for such an unconscionably long period of time?

He was bombarded endlessly with questions about his original examination of the patient. What did he actually feel? What didn't he feel? What might he have felt? What should he have felt? And if he had felt nothing, what was his explanation for this "error?" Why did he not perform a full biopsy of the area in question?

In truth, Bush was guilty of none of these charges of neglect or incompetence. Given the rarity of breast cancer among women of this age, there was only a small segment of them in whom any concern at all might be justified, and closer tracking maintained. There was a need to follow closely any of those with a suspicious mass, but this was not found by either of the two experienced doctors who had examined Mary.

In the absence of such objective evidence, some women are at a higher risk of developing breast cancer at an early age and might merit closer observation than ordinary. If, for example, a woman has her first pregnancy relatively late in her reproductive life, then she is believed to be more susceptible to breast cancer; Mary had had her first pregnancy in her twenties. Smoking, alcohol, and obesity had all been implicated as risk factors. Mary neither smoked, drank, nor had ever had any weight problems. As for performing a full surgical biopsy of the area in question, this was not only unnecessary, but slashing open a woman's breast for tissue samples without justification in itself would have constituted a grave commission of malpractice.

Much was made by the plaintiff's lawyer about the aunt with breast cancer, despite, as has already been noted, the lack of risk associated with this kind of kinship. The lawyer, nevertheless, continued to hammer away at it.

Q. Were you aware of the fact that Mrs. Parker's aunt had died from breast cancer?

A. Yes, I was.

Q. And you attached no importance to this?

A. No, I did not. There is no statistical evidence supporting an increased risk of breast cancer in a woman with an aunt who has had the disease.

Q. How about two aunts?

A. The same would probably apply.

Q. Well how about three aunts or four aunts?

A. Yes, I suppose that would cause me to think about it. So would five or six aunts!

Q. Even if the mother and any sisters were not affected?

A. I suppose so.

Q. I trust we can assume that the answer to that question is "yes."

The seed had been planted in the minds of the jury. It certainly seemed possible that *some* weight should have been given to the fact that Mary's aunt had died from the disease.

Another item that caused Bush trouble was the drawing he had sent with Mary on her first visit to Vera. It showed a breast with an arrow pointing to the area in question. Bush's intent was to indicate the area about which the patient was concerned. The plaintiff's lawyer kept suggesting that it was the area in which Bush, himself, had felt a suspicious mass.

Perhaps most damaging to Bush in regard to the initial episode was the act of aspirating the breast area to which the patient referred even though he could feel nothing there. This was certainly a minor, harmless procedure, taking only a minute or two to attempt sucking some cells and tissue fluid back into the small syringe. It had been done primarily for the purpose of reassuring the patient. The gynecologist appearing as an expert witness for the plaintiff completely torpedoed this explanation by testifying that there was no indication for a physician to aspirate a breast unless he or she had identified a specific mass within the breast. The implication here was clearly that if Bush had performed an aspiration, by this very act he certainly must have felt the mass of which the patient had complained, and should have proceeded to a full surgical biopsy following the negative findings obtained from the needle aspiration.

As Vera prepared to give testimony in her own defense, the same questions asserted themselves to her over and over. "Why am I here? What in the world ever possessed them to accuse me, of all people?" Her physical examination of the patient had not been criticized. There had been no objections concerning her interpretation of the mammograms. Her reading of the films seemed to have been accepted as completely valid, as they indeed were. At no point during the trial were any of her interpretations of the films challenged.

As for all that hokum about blood spurting from the breast as an early sign of cancer, this could easily be looked upon as simply a straw man put up by the opposition, one that a spirited defense could easily topple. As for the need for follow-up mammograms, even when some abnormality is suspected— which in this case it was not—the standard is to wait three to six months because it takes this long ordinarily for detectible changes to occur. Mary had returned in four months.

But when the plaintiff's radiologist held her culpable *if* the blood spurting advice was the only warning given and Vera's attorney just seemed to leave it at that, and when other charges against her seemed to pass through the courtroom hardly deflected by the defense on their way to the jury, her fears grew.

The issue concerning the decision not to use ultrasound after the first mammogram was relentlessly pursued by Mary's attorney. Never mind that ultrasound was much less sensitive than mammography in detecting breast cancers and that it was used only to determine the character of the contents within a mass already demonstrated on mammography or physical examination.

Q. Did you have an ultrasound machine available to you?

A. Yes, across the street in the hospital.

Q. Did you ever use it in patients with suspected breast cancer?

A. Yes.

Q. Is it a painful procedure for the patient to undergo?

A. No.

Q. Is it particularly expensive?

A. No.

Q. Are there any unpleasant side effects from ultrasound?

A. No.

Q. Then why, in a patient who insisted that a new mass had appeared in her breast, as indeed it had, did you refuse to perform such a simple, harmless and inexpensive procedure that might have helped make the diagnosis?

Vera's logical explanation seemed to fall on deaf ears. And as the trial wore on and Mary's attorney began to question not only Vera's competence but her integrity as well, any feelings about the unassailability of her position vanished completely. If not a straw man, perhaps it was a straw cross that the opposition was constructing, one that, its flimsy construction notwithstanding, might still well serve for Vera's professional crucifixion.

After testimony concerning the alleged failure of the defendants to make the proper diagnosis in a timely manner, the trial began to focus on the next major consideration of the malpractice action. Given the fact that the diagnosis was not made until four months after the patient originally presented herself in Bush's office, what harm did this delay represent to the patient in terms of her chances for survival?

The judge and jury were now about to undergo a crash course about prognosticating cancer, breast cancer especially, Mary Parker's breast cancer in particular.

Given the propensity for many cancers to recur following initial treatment, cancer specialists (oncologists) are reluctant to talk about cures. They refer, instead, to five- or ten-year survival rates in the absence of recurrence. Early diagnosis, detecting cancer in its initial stages, has generally offered the best chance for successful therapy, and the technique of staging is used to predict the likelihood of successful treatment of just about all cancers. Size of the neoplasm at the time of discovery, extent of spread, histological appearance of the cancer cells under the microscope, and other factors all contribute to the estimation of chances for success or failure of treatment; the earlier the stage at the time of discovery, the better the chance for long-term survival.

In breast cancer, Stage I signifies that the cancer discovered is less than two centimeters (three quarters of an inch) in size and limited to the breast, with no involvement of the lymph nodes draining the breast. Stage II signifies that the neoplasm is between two and five centimeters in its largest dimension with or without clinically suspected lymph node involvement. Stage III is reserved for those with cancers larger than five centimeters in size and with definite overlying skin involvement or spread to the axillary nodes. Stage IV includes those patients with distant spread (metastases) to areas such as the bone, brain, or lung.

In Mary's case, as might well have been expected, the attorneys for the plaintiff and defendants presented quite different scenarios regarding her status when she first appeared and then four months later. No one denied that she had cancer, whatever the size and extent, when she initially appeared, although it was probably under two centimeters in size, the ordinary threshold of palpability by examining physicians. The size four months later was, however, a major problem for even the most objective of observers. With the use of the ultrasound image, the plaintiff's attorneys claimed that it was 5.4 centimeters in its major dimension. The size, as determined by the pathologist, who measured it directly following its surgical removal, was reported as 5.0 centimeters. Using the ultrasonic value, this would have put the patient clearly into Stage III; using the direct anatomical measurement put the patient clearly in limbo, somewhere between Stage II and Stage III.

At the time of surgery, one axillary lymph node was found to have been positive for cancer cells. According to the plaintiff's oncologist this had occurred during the four-month interim from the first visit to the second. This would mean that the patient had progressed from a Stage I breast cancer to a Stage III. The oncologist for the defense contended that, in all probability, given the rapid progression of the tumor, the lymph node had most likely been involved at the time of the first visit. In short, he contended that no real progression in stage had occurred.

The defense oncologist also stressed some aspects of pathology that might not have been readily appreciated by the lay persons constituting the jury. First was the microscopic appearance of the cancer. The more organized or near normal in structure the cancer cell, the better the outlook for success in treating the patient. In Mary's case the cells were highly disorganized ("undifferentiated") in appearance, boding ill for future survival right from the beginning. The other question involved with prognosis was the absence of so-called estrogen receptors on the tumor cells. If these were present, then anti-estrogen therapy might have been effective in prolonging survival. As is the case with most young women with breast cancer, such was not the case with Mary.

In summary, the oncological staging of the neoplasm was from Stage I to Stage III four months later according to the plaintiff's attorneys. The defense argued that it was already Stage III, albeit on a microscopic scale, when Mary first appeared in Dr. Bush's office. The plaintiff's attorneys maintained that as a result of a four-month delay in treatment, the five-year survival probability had diminished from 90 percent to about 20 percent. The defense maintained that a ten-year survival estimate was more realistic and that the reduction in survival for this period as a result of delay in treatment could not have amounted to more than 35 percent at most instead of the 70 percent postulated by the plaintiff.

Whatever the truth of the matter, if any truth could be approximated on purely scientific grounds, as far as any juror might be concerned in the highly charged atmosphere surrounding the proceedings, it was more of a crying game than a numbers game in which they were involved. Mary had been divorced from her husband a year before her illness had taken hold and was contemplating a new marriage with a young man with whom she had fallen in love and who had ardently returned her affection, winning that of the two little girls as well. When he was called to the stand to testify about his own knowledge of his fiancée's illness and the effects it had had upon their relationship, he began to sob uncontrollably.

The courtroom was rather small and of an unusual configuration, one which placed the spectators and jury in unusually clear sight of one another. Throughout the trial Mary's parents and even those of her former husband, still deeply attached to Mary, sat day after day in the courtroom, the agony, sadness, and frequent anger of their faces constantly in view of the jurors. Frequently, throughout the trial, many eyes were filled with tears as the tragedy of the young woman's illness unfolded. Perhaps the only person who did not succumb to this was Mary herself. As she sat in the witness box, frail, wasted, and obviously in some pain, her head covered with a turban to hide the hair loss due to chemotherapy, she stoically related the suffering she had endured, including the other side effects of her chemotherapy such as almost constant nausea, weakness, and other debilitating symptoms over an eight-month period when she was unable to work. She spoke of the growing chest pain she was experiencing after the cancer had spread to her lung. She mentioned her applications to be included in the bone marrow replacement trials, which, thus far, had gone unanswered. She spoke of her fading hopes for a future marriage. Most of all, she expressed her anxieties about her two little girls and how they might be cared for in the event of her death, which now seemed more imminent with the passage of every day.

Through all this testimony Mary remained clear-eyed, but no one else did. Not her lover, her parents, the jury, the spectators, nor Vera, who, at this point, despite her convictions about her complete innocence in the matter, would not have denied this courageous young woman some recompense for her tragic condition.

Following adjournment on the final day of Mary's testimony, Vera's attorney approached her with a recommendation for settlement out of court. They both knew now that the jury was almost certainly sure to go against them. For Vera, financial considerations began to loom ever more prominent in her thinking. Although she had coverage up to three million dollars through several policies, she faced the possibility of even greater damages if this was left to a jury. Multimillion-dollar awards were rare but they did happen; one read of them in the newspapers every day, and in cases much less heartrending than this one. What if the judgment against her exceeded the three million? Would she and her husband lose their home? Would they have to turn over all their savings? Would they be able to continue financing the educations of their three children then in college?

Vera decided to agree to this course of action, and although the superficial justification for this was a financial one, deep down within her she could not escape a feeling of guilt at having failed her patient and even a desire to be punished in some way, regardless of the facts of the case. A settlement was made within the confines of her coverage, and her connection with subsequent events was severed.

Jim Bush persisted to the end, and Vera could only surmise

all his reasons for doing so. This had not been the first case brought against him, unjustified in his eyes, and he was still smarting from previous instances of alleged malpractice of which he had ultimately been found innocent. Indeed, frequent malpractice suits had become part and parcel of all obstetrical-gynecological practices as patient demands for perfection had become routine in the preceding decades of increasing litigation. But, as sympathetic as he was to the plight of Mary, he was enraged at what he considered the betrayal of a patient with whom he thought he had established such good rapport and devotion. No doubt he felt deeply that his exoneration should be complete and public. This was not to be. The case concluded, not surprisingly, in favor of the plaintiff. Vera and Bush were found guilty in their failure to diagnose and treat the patient properly. The amount awarded was three million dollars, levied equally upon them.

Having settled for considerably less before the end of the trial, Vera had no further financial responsibilities. But Jim Bush's insurance inadequately covered the penalty against him. Bush and his attorneys immediately brought a motion for a mistrial.

The judge's perception of the way the trial had gone was, of course, critical to this decision, and his written comments about the trial revealed his own misgivings from the outset. Any trial, by its very nature, is adversarial and likely to contain a good deal of finger-pointing and vituperation. In a case of alleged medical malpractice, especially one concerning a young mother at death's door, such aspects in the proceedings had been inescapable. The judge had been aware of this from the start, but had hoped to get through the trial with both sides treated fairly. He had been especially concerned about the physical proximity of the jury to the courtroom spectators, mostly Mary's relatives and friends.

The lawyer representing Mary inescapably must have been aware of this but refused to be satisfied with this technical advantage alone. From the beginning he adopted a strategy to vilify the defendants and draw them only in the harshest light to the jury. The first step along these lines involved jury selection.

Mary Matsuoko had been born in California. Her grandparents had immigrated from Tokyo. She was, therefore, a third-generation American and as equal in her claim to nationality as most of those in the courtroom. "Parker" was the name of her former husband. As prospective jurors were polled, the judge, much to his later regret, had allowed the attorneys for the plaintiff to include an inappropriate question: Do you believe those of Oriental background or descent to be any more or less trustworthy than others? The suggestions that because of her racial background she was treated by her doctors in a less proper manner than might otherwise have been the case increased in frequency and intensity, despite frequent objections from the defense.

The trial had been a long and arduous one. When the time for summations finally arrived, in order to conclude them expeditiously, the judged had instructed the defense lawyers from withholding any objections to the plaintiff's lawyers' presentation throughout its course. This opened the door to another legal excursion by the plaintiff's lawyer, one that ventured well beyond any bounds of ethical courtroom propriety. Bush and Vera were characterized as "fancy" [read "white"] doctors who had ignored the problems of a minority single mother. They were also charged with concocting their stories, trying to "con" the jury, and in essence being guilty of collusion when, in truth, the only contact about the case between Bush and Vera had been a phone call from Bush, who had already received his notification, the day before Vera received her own summons to ask if she was to be involved as well.

Finally, it was the actions of the jury itself that convinced the judge to declare a mistrial. Both sides had agreed that Mary had been afflicted with cancer from the very beginning; in the judge's words, "it was not as if the defendants had caused the cancer." Yet in their awarding of damages, the jury had acted as if Mary would have had a 100 percent cure if the doctors had acted differently from the very start, a position not even the most biased of observers could logically maintain. The judge simply could not allow this to stand.

Details about subsequent events came to Vera secondhand. She learned that a new trial for Jim Bush had been scheduled but that he finally decided to settle out of court before it had begun.

Additional chemotherapy did not help Mary, and given the particulars of the experimental trials of bone marrow transplantation for breast cancer at various research centers, Mary had failed to qualify for any of them. She died a year later, shortly before her thirty-eighth birthday.

One thinks of winners and losers at a trial, but it was difficult to think of anyone who had really won here. As a result of the ordeal, Vera's self-confidence was severely shaken. Her group had an ultrasound unit installed in their offices in a room immediately adjacent to the mammography unit. A good many more ultrasound studies were now being performed on women in conjunction with mammography for suspected breast cancer, a number of them probably with questionable scientific justification, but undoubtedly increasing the cost of medical care. Because of the potential for later litigation on the basis of physical findings, many radiologists, including those in her group, had begun to refuse performing breast examinations even though they might prove helpful in performing and interpreting the mammographic studies and possibly confirming the referring doctor's findings or not. After all, such radiologists could maintain, their job was to take X-rays and not to perform physicals on patients or advise them about their future medical management.

Although Vera felt an obligation to continue examining these women herself, she did so with the knowledge that any one of them might turn into a legal adversary. She continued to reassure when she could but, with the memory of her ordeal in court, was unable to do so as effectively as was the case before her devastating trial.

Jim Bush finally surrendered to despair. Although still youthful and vigorous at the conclusion of the trial, he had lost his zest for medical practice and retired five to ten years earlier than might otherwise have been the case, bitter to the end at the perceived injustices inflicted upon him.

Mary's lover had lost the wife he had hoped would share the rest of his life with him. Her parents had lost a daughter, their only child. Her children had lost a loving mother. And Mary had lost her life.

No simple winners and losers here, only victims. Victims all.

12

THE END OF THE ROAD

A DOCTOR AND HIS PATIENT TRY TO GROW OLD TOGETHER

My mother, for as long as she lived, never ever was convinced that I had become a *real* doctor. To her way of thinking, a real doctor had a busy office, hundreds upon hundreds of grateful, worshipful private patients, a big house, an almost bigger car, and a whopping bank account to support them.

I know it was something of a disappointment to her when I spent most of my early professional life in the animal laboratory. I lived in small studio apartments; my cars were all economy-size and for a long time secondhand; and about all the patients I saw were poverty-stricken ones in hospital clinics. There was some truth in her perception of what a doctor should be and one which, to some extent, I shared with her. I entered medical school fully intending to become a general practitioner, later deciding upon internal medicine. Either kind of practice involves what we now call primary care, directed at forming a lasting intimate relationship with one's patients and their families in addition to administering to their health needs. However, by the time I had finished my residency training in internal medicine, I had become enamored with cardiology and soon after undertook a fellowship in cardiovascular diseases. Bitten by the research bug, I gravitated into a career of academic medicine, emphasizing teaching and laboratory investigation, far removed from the kind of career both my mother and I had originally envisioned for me.

Dorothy Z. was one of the few exceptions to my subsequent pattern of practice. For more than twenty years I enjoyed and suffered through with her all that the idealized doctor-patient relationship entails.

Despite my position on the faculty of a medical school, among my duties was to devote half a day each week for consultative services to various patients with cardiac problems referred to us by local practitioners. It was in this capacity that I originally saw Dorothy in Jersey City when our medical school was still called the Seton Hall College of Medicine and before we moved to Newark and became the New Jersey Medical School, part of the University of Medicine and Dentistry of New Jersey.

It was in 1968 and Dorothy, at forty, was exactly the same age as I. For the previous two years she had suffered increased symptoms of palpitation and shortness of breath. She recalled having had rheumatic fever as a child, and now it was catching up with her in the guise of rheumatic heart disease. Although this occurs in less than 5 percent of those who have had rheumatic fever, Dorothy was one of the unlucky ones, and it would place her in my care for the next twenty-one years. To understand what went wrong and occasionally right with Dorothy, you must first understand just a little of the anatomy and function of the normal heart.

Four chambers of the heart can be described, two composing the right side and two the left side of this organ. A thin-walled right atrium receives all the venous blood from various parts of the body and delivers it to a muscular-walled right ventricle, which pumps it out through the pulmonary artery to the lungs for oxygenation. From the lungs the blood is delivered to the left atrium, similar in structure to its partner on the right, and then is transmitted to the muscular left ventricle, which pumps it through the large arterial vessel, the aorta, and its branches throughout the body. Strategically placed valves within the heart ensure that the blood flows only in a forward direction. The tricuspid valve prevents backflow from the right ventricle to the right atrium, and the pulmonic valve prevents backflow from the pulmonary artery to the right ventricle. On the left side of the heart the mitral valve, situated between the left atrium and left ventricle, similarly prevents the backflow of blood from the ventricle to the atrium as it contracts to force blood out into the aorta. The aortic valve acts similarly to the pulmonic valve in preventing backflow into the ventricle as the heart finishes a contraction and begins to relax prior to the next beat.

Rheumatic fever, when it affects the heart, involves all parts of it, including the walls of the chambers and even the sac around the heart, the pericardium. But clinically it is the valves that usually take the brunt of the attack as the disease smolders on, unnoticed by the victim for many years until symptoms appear and bring about a visit to the doctor's office. The chronic inflammatory process and the scarring that follows it result in a deforming of one or more valves that might result in prevention of their opening normally (stenosis) or closing properly (regurgitation). Sometimes a combination of these malfunctions occurs, with the valve being neither able to open nor close properly (combined stenosis and regurgitation).

In Dorothy's case, it was the most common scenario of those with rheumatic heart disease: the mitral valve between the left atrium and ventricle had become narrowed or stenotic, and the blood, unable to pass normally from atrium to ventricle, was backing up into her lungs, causing congestion and breathlessness. This became immediately apparent to me as I listened over the left lower portion of the chest in this tall, ungainly, pale woman who was putting up a brave front despite the severity of her symptoms. There I heard the ominous rumbling murmur of mitral stenosis as the insufficient eddies of blood attempted passage through the narrowed valve. It turned out that there was some aortic valve leaking or regurgitation, but this was not deemed critical at the time. A heart catheterization confirmed these impressions, and fortunately we had a remedy to offer: open heart surgery.

Since Dorothy's problem was in essence a mechanical one, by opening of the valve manually under direct vision with open heart surgery or replacing it with an artificial valve, the surgeon could restore a normal or nearly normal opening and relieve the symptoms that had incapacitated her. The operation was successfully performed on her mitral valve without the need for valve replacement. With the surgical part of her treatment accomplished, the rest was up to me.

I mentioned palpitations, a sensation related to an irregular heartbeat, that had also troubled Dorothy. This particular irregularity, atrial fibrillation, is common in patients with rheumatic heart disease. In essence, the atria, instead of beating regularly seventy or eighty times per minute as in normal hearts, develop a rapid kind of twitching activity that is ineffective in propagating the normal electrical impulses to the ventricles for their own beating. As a result, the ventricles, although beating much slower than the atria, are activated to contract in an irregular way, often causing the perception of thumping within the chest of the patient. Converting atrial fibrillation to normal rhythm by medication or electric shock is often tried but often fails to persist. However, as long as the overall ventricular rate is fairly normal, the pumping function of the heart can be maintained. The major problem with atrial fibrillation lies in the atria, especially the left atrium, where within the low-flow dilated chamber blood clots (thrombi) can form. When portions of these break loose they can be ejected out the aorta and travel widely throughout the body to any vital organ (thromboembolism). Often they reach arteries to the brain, and these so-called emboli can occur in as many as one out of five patients with atrial fibrillation resulting from rheumatic heart disease. The likelihood becomes ever greater with the passage of time. Such episodes can be severely incapacitating or even fatal. The only solution, if conversion back to normal rhythm is unsuccessful, is to anticoagulate the patient for the duration to prevent such clots from ever forming.

My initial encounters with Dorothy convinced me that,

whatever I attempted to achieve in treating her, it would demand of me all the powers of persuasion and tact that I could muster. Noted for my own "short fuse," I soon found Dorothy's to be even shorter. I suppose we would call her something other than a spinster today, but that is what she was then. She had lived with her aging parents all her life in Jersey City. Her mother was a big red-faced woman whose head was topped by a gray bun, but whose quiet demeanor belied her florid appearance. Dorothy's father was a rather shadowy figure who died shortly after Dorothy came under my care; I never met him.

As far as I could surmise, Dorothy did not have much of a social life. She worked as a bookkeeper for a local business where the absences occasioned by her illness were not well received, complicating her response to therapy. But more of this later.

I started with attempting to convert her cardiac rhythm back to normal even though I had no illusions about how successful I might be. If the atrial fibrillation is of recent onset—no more than a few weeks in duration, for example—the restoration of normal rhythm is often achieved. In Dorothy's case, where the disordered rhythm had probably been in place for at least a year before her surgery, the chances of such success were slim, but at least it was worth a try. Electrical cardioversion (administering electric shocks through the chest wall with paddles applied to the chest of the sedated patient) in combination with drugs eventually failed. As for the drugs I prescribed, Dorothy tended to develop just about every side effect described for them, necessitating their ultimate withdrawal. Needless to add, she held me personally responsible for the effects these poisonous substances were having on her and, I suppose, in a sense she was justified, although they were all we had to work with.

Stymied by attempts to convert the heart rhythm back to normal, I decided to rely on anticoagulation. Here there was greater hope for success, since medications prescribed to "thin the blood" were of proved effectiveness in many thousands of patients so treated and reported in the medical literature. Unfortunately, Dorothy was not one of them. No matter how carefully I titrated the dosages of the medications to maintain her within the therapeutic range, her blood-clotting tests revealed that she was either inadequately treated or excessively anticoagulated and in danger of severe bleeding. In fact she had to be admitted to the hospital for two severe bleeding episodes, but both were controlled without causing permanent damage. After the second of these Dorothy refused any further attempts at anticoagulation, and I was hard put to disagree. We would have to take our chances in the future in regard to the threat of thromboembolism. Miraculously, not one instance of thromboembolism occurred over the next two decades. But other problems would arise.

Although the surgery had been an unqualified success in relieving the mitral valve obstruction, Dorothy continued complaining about fatigue, chest pains, shortness of breath, and a variety of other complaints each time she visited me. The reason for these complaints eventually became apparent to me. It was not her heart that was her problem but her supervisor at work. He strongly resented every hour she was absent and made no secret of this through his constant harassment in the office.

Although I have always maintained that continued productive employment, if at all possible, is one of the best therapies for patients, I finally gave in and arranged for Dorothy to receive total disability payments from the Social Security Administration. Such an act on my part was not entirely fraudulent. Contrary to popular belief, most patients who undergo major heart valve surgery in adult life do not hop off the operating table and begin training for the next Olympics. The residue of wear and tear visited upon their hearts over the preceding years often requires drug therapy and constant observation over many years.

In Dorothy's case the psychological effects of being freed from the tyranny of her supervisor were remarkable. Most of the post-operative complaints either disappeared or were minimized within a very short time.

Without the need for frequent visits to monitor her anticoagulant therapy, our encounters fell off from biweekly to monthly and then to quarterly intervals. She would appear in my office, feisty as ever in the company of her fawning mother, and invariably bawl me out whenever my stethoscope pressed too firmly along the sensitized portion of her scar—exactly, of course, in the location I was required to listen to make a valid judgment. And woe betide me if I was ever late for a visit! I learned to be prompt, thanks to her scolding, and gradually earned a reputation among my other patients as that rare bird, a doctor who was often in the examining room well ahead of his patients, awaiting their arrival.

Over the next few years Dorothy managed to outlive the local GP who had initially referred her to me. She then outlasted his successor, who would not or could not handle her. She informed me that from then on I was to be her sole doctor, like it or not. When the medical school moved to Newark, and I with it, she followed me into Essex County, although she never failed to complain about the traffic from Jersey City or the inadequate parking facilities that I (!) had provided for her.

She did well for a remarkably long time. Although the findings of the leaking aortic valve (aortic regurgitation) became a bit more prominent with the improved blood flow following relief of the mitral stenosis, I had no doubts about her being able to tolerate this for an extended period. We continued our habitual good-natured barking at one another over the years, and I assured Dorothy that we would grow old and ornery together. I hoped that such light banter would conceal from her my greatest fears: that one day a clot would form in the left atrium and embolize, as was often the case with such patients; or that the effects of the valve-widening at surgery would wear off in time and significant narrowing once again occur.

By 1982, thirteen years following her surgery, I was convinced that the mitral stenosis had recurred and now, with recently introduced echocardiographic techniques (ultrasound) I could fairly estimate just how small the opening was. To confirm this I suggested another heart catheterization, but Dorothy refused. She felt fine, she told me, although I suspected that, like many cardiac patients in such circumstances, she was severely limiting her physical activity in order to minimize any symptoms that might otherwise be induced.

Incredibly this tug of war went on between us for the next seven years, perhaps suggesting that Dorothy really did know more about her disease than her doctor. But by 1990 she could no longer beat the odds, which by now had piled up against her immeasurably. On her regular visit, as I listened over her chest I noticed that in addition to the findings of severe mitral stenosis, the whooshing sound of the leaking aortic valve had been replaced by the unnerving harsh hiss of aortic stenosis. The aortic valve, over time, had been converted by the chronic scarring and calcification from a moderately leaking one to a severely obstructed one. Unlike aortic regurgitation, aortic stenosis carries with it the risk of sudden death. In addition to this, a third valve, the tricuspid on the right side of the heart between the right atrium and ventricle, had begun to leak severely. I implored her to come to the hospital for further evaluation and surgery. She said she would think about it and retreated to Jersey City.

A week later an ambulance delivered her to the emergency room in severe congestive heart failure. She finally agreed to the second operation, at which time the surgeon found it necessary to replace all three of the affected valves. It was just too much for her to tolerate. Post-operatively her kidneys failed, her lungs failed, her blood clotting failed, and her heart failed as a result of an overwhelming infection. She was sixty-one.

I agonized over whether or not I should have been more insistent about the mitral surgery seven years earlier. Perhaps with this taken care of she would have been able to survive later on the additional surgery required by the other two involved valves. This and other questions about alternative choices that might have been made continued to haunt me in the aftermath of her death.

I wrote to her widowed mother, now alone in her eighties. I expressed to her all the affection I had developed for her daughter, for whom I had cared for longer than any other patient in my years as a physician. I told the mother how much I had wished that Dorothy and I could really have grown old instead of just older together as doctor and patient.

Perhaps I could have written of this experience to my own mother if she was still alive. Perhaps she would have finally relented and admitted that, deep down under all that professorial veneer, I had been a real doctor after all.

13

MODERN MEDICINE

A CASE OF FALLING SHORT

Reba Jackson was a twenty-three-year-old African American mother of four preschool children without a man in the house and totally dependent upon welfare agencies for subsistence. This was not an unusual set of circumstances for a young black woman transplanted from the South to the Newark of the 1970s.

Early one May morning there was, however, a more unusual component added to the picture. As her children attempted to awaken her from sleep, she lay in bed semi-comatose, unable to speak and with one-half of her body paralyzed. She had had a cerebral embolism. Although she would be found to have a cardiac condition similar to that of Dorothy Z., the course of her disease, its treatment, and the outcome were strikingly different.

For many years Reba had known that she had something called "a rheumatic heart," but as time went on she gradually reduced the level of her daily activities so as to avoid the spells of palpitation and shortness of breath that would otherwise occur. The mitral valve of the heart had become severely narrowed (mitral stenosis) and she had developed atrial fibrillation. This was the perfect setting for clot formation in the enlarged left atrium and predisposition toward possible thromboembolism when part or all of the clot can break loose from the inner wall of the atrium. When this finally did occur, the clot traversed the valve into the left ventricle, went out the aorta, and lodged in an arterial branch supplying an important part of her brain. It was the area that controlled movements of the right side of the body. Had she been slightly less unfortunate the clot may have gone to an arm or leg where the abrupt cut-off of blood flow would simply have resulted in sudden cold and pain in the affected extremity. This could soon be remedied by surgical removal of the clot from the artery involved. In the brain no such operation was possible, and Reba stood as high as a 25 percent chance of dying from the insult.

The medical response of the hospital was prompt. The diagnosis was obvious on admission, and within weeks the patient's condition was stabilized enough to permit open heart surgery to replace the diseased valve with an artificial one. Post-operatively the response of the heart was satisfactory, but the effects of the brain damage were still devastating. In addition to the nearly total right-sided paralysis, she was unable to speak. She maintained some control over the muscles of speech, and she understood what was said to her, but due to the damage of the motor center for speech she was unable to respond: an expressive aphasia.

It was imperative to transfer her as soon as possible to one of the several centers in the county where the work of rehabilitation could begin, but it was now that the oppressive weight of the social system began to be felt. For no known reason some minor functionary at a city or state department had removed Reba from the Medicaid program, under which the costs of rehabilitation would be paid. She had been transferred to another program that did not provide this benefit. The rehabilitation centers that were approached refused to accept her without some guarantee of payment. Once the bureaucratic wheel had turned, it seemed that there was no reversing it and getting her reassigned to Medicaid. The social worker as well as the doctors caring for her tried every means of persuasion: cajoling, pleading, and threatening, all to no avail.

Such is the nature of the neuromuscular damage following any stroke that each day of rehabilitation lost early in the course of recovery often results in deformity and disability that may take weeks to reverse at a later date. The necessary facilities and personnel at the busy city hospital were inadequate to the task as the overworked and understaffed nursing department could do little to supplement them. As the months of inaction passed, the muscles of Reba's shoulder girdle atrophied and resulted in a dislocation requiring orthopedic surgical treatment.

With the limited physical therapy the hospital was able to offer, Reba did finally manage to stand but was unable to walk or speak. By midwinter it was clear that the game was up. After more than seven months following hospital admission and after more than six months since the successful heart surgery, Reba was returned home to join her children, still speechless and unable to walk without assistance. It was December 24. Merry Christmas.*

---

* Easter was merrier. By March of the new year efforts to have her restored to the Medicaid program finally succeeded and physical rehabilitation treatments were begun.

14

THE SURVIVOR

THE STRANGE AND UNPREDICTABLE QUALITIES
OF PERSONALITY THAT ALLOWED A PATIENT TO
RISE ABOVE HIS DISEASE AND HOW IT WON
THE GRUDGING RESPECT OF HIS DOCTOR

I first met JJ on morning rounds. He was presented to me by my medical resident as one of the new admissions of the day. He was a ruggedly handsome black man of medium height and build with a well-trimmed moustache and a ready smile. He sported a purple bandanna on his head, knotted in the back a bit to the side, pirate-style. He looked much younger than his forty-four years and his body, in general, was in magnificent shape, the kind you see on parallel bar gymnasts. What made it all so grotesque were the forearms, swollen Popeye-like from the thousands of needles that had penetrated the skin over a lifetime of drug abuse.

It was not these, however, that had led to his hospital admission. Rather it was a mild fever and a slightly painful swelling in the right upper arm under the biceps. We thought he might be at the early stages of a potentially serious infection. Blood cultures were drawn, and he was started on an appropriate antibiotic regimen. A CT (computed tomography) scan had been ordered so that the area of involvement might better be delineated. Our surgeons were notified and asked to take a look and consider the advisability of open drainage.

Although his arm was causing some discomfort, this was not JJ's major concern that morning. He had full dentures and somehow during the previous night his lowers had split right down the middle into two halves. He was having considerable difficulty keeping them in place so that he could chew solid food properly.

He had tried to join the two halves together with some ordinary paste and was still engaged in this fruitless effort when we approached the bedside. Before we had left it we had ascertained the various possibilities regarding his arm; we had also become aware of the dental problem, implored by the patient to have something done about it.

My resident had already called the dental department but,

knowing how slowly they usually responded, especially to problems of this sort, I advised JJ not to have too high hopes of a quick resolution to his predicament. I reckoned that they would either simply give him an appointment for the dental clinic upon his discharge or, at least, take the denture for repair and *perhaps* JJ would be lucky enough to get it back intact within two to three weeks' time.

"If only I had some Crazy Glue," JJ thought aloud, "that might do it."

At that moment the imaginary lightbulb of an idea lit up over my head. What a wonderful opportunity to demonstrate to my medical students and house staff what it meant to be a *real* doctor. So often the complaint with which a patient enters a hospital turns out to have nothing to do with what we uncover to be the real risk to his life or well-being. ("So what if he does have a toothache? It's the possible brain tumor that has to be investigated!")

However, the patient does not forget the toothache, and as this complaint becomes lost in the maelstrom of all our medical activities, diagnostic and otherwise, we risk alienating the subject of our concern and losing his confidence and cooperation. I would not make such a mistake this time, I vowed. Without informing my assistants of my plan, I obtained some Crazy Glue at home that night and brought it to the hospital the next morning. I had little hope that it would repair the denture, but was confident that it would certainly cement the proper doctor-patient relationship I wished to demonstrate. Mission accomplished!

Pleased as punch with myself, I led my retinue to JJ's room. We entered to find him shadow-boxing against one wall. The antibiotics were obviously having some effect in helping his arm along.

"I've got the glue," I exulted, taking the tube from my pocket and thrusting it before him.

This was met with a broad and complete smile, uppers and lowers intact. "Hey, Doc. No need for that now. I got the real thing—a professional job."

True to form, the staff dentist had acted as I predicted. What I did not foresee was that he had his own retinue of students and that JJ had somehow managed to corral one or two of these to run off to their laboratory and perform a quick repair job for him the same day.

This was no ordinary "hophead" I was dealing with, and I must admit I had to admire how skillfully he had managed to manipulate the system to his advantage. I resolved to talk with him in another role, that of the personal interviewer, inquiring about his lifestyle and experiences outside the fringes of normal society. JJ graciously acquiesced to my request, and a day later he lay back in bed, arms folded behind his head, to field any questions that I might put to him.

He informed me that he had actually been born in Maryland but that at the age of three he had moved with his family to the Newark area—Orange, New Jersey, to be precise. He attributed most of his early troubles to lead poisoning. This, he explained, was due to exposure to a contaminated sand pit in which he played and which "messed up" his scalp. Although ringworm was a likelier diagnosis, I let it go. I suspect that even JJ, with his limited education, knew the truth, but the fiction he had constructed for himself just fit that much better into the persona that seemed to work best for him.

Although he never graduated from high school, it was there that he found he was pretty handy with his fists. A mayoral program he identified as "Outward Bound" led to his becoming an amateur featherweight, with frequent tours around the country over a ten-year period. I inquired if he had ever fought professionally.

"Oh no," he assured me, "my profession is shoplifting."

I probed for details.

"Well, I deal mainly in TV sets, microwaves, refrigerators, electronics—stuff like that."

I could not envision him walking around department stores and concealing something like a large television set under his raincoat. He enlightened me.

"I don't go into no store, Doc. I go to platforms. You know, you buy something inside and then pick it up on the back platform. All I do is pick it up before the customer does. That's how I got this here hernia once when I picked up a refrigerator." He pointed to a scar in his groin. I was somehow relieved to learn that there was no violence involved with all of this.

"I been locked up twenty-four times for shoplifting"—it sounded like an item on his expense account—"but busted only once for H and B [housebreaking and burglary] but that was a bum rap. The other dude had stolen *my* microwave and VCR and then told the police that I had stolen it from *him*."

I wondered how he had gotten into drugs. According to JJ, it was the threat of induction and going to Vietnam that started it. "Man, I just walked in there higher than a kite. The gave me a 1Y and I was out of it."

I doubted that it was simply an appointment with Selective Service that had initiated him into the use of drugs, but I wondered about that 1Y classification. Yes, there still is a Selective Service office operating in Washington, and I called for enlightenment. They tried to be helpful. It seems that the true meaning of "1Y" has changed over time and with different administrations. I gathered finally that it sort of meant that if the entire country was on the verge of sliding off the continental shelf they might just consider calling in the 1Ys for some assistance.

The drug use had continued for more than two decades, and although JJ was on methadone now, I doubted whether the heroin and all the rest had ever completely ceased. Somehow he had also managed to get onto Social Security's total disability list. In JJ's word, "They pay me to be a good boy."

Although this could not have amounted to a great deal of money, he assured me that he didn't have to buy anything and proudly lifted the lapel of the Bill Blass silk robe he was wearing.

What about family, a wife, children? There was no wife in his life, but four loving women. They must have been loving, at least in one sense, because they provided him with a total of fifteen children: fourteen girls and one boy. "He's the puny one," JJ laughed. He told me that the women still came to visit him in the hospital.

As the days of hospitalization wore on, the swelling under his biceps subsided, as did the fever. Whatever the original problem was, it seemed to be resolving, and JJ was anxious to get back home to "collect his rents." I did not pursue this. Perhaps he had lifted an apartment off some loading dock along with all those refrigerators and TVs.

As he was about to leave the hospital, he had a final request. He asked us to arrange for a homemaker to be sent to him several times a week to help him out. Him, with four wives and fourteen daughters!

"Doc, I can't even cook an egg," he protested.

This was a bit much for me at this stage. "A homemaker? JJ, we send homemakers to people who cannot even get out of bed, people who are paralyzed from the neck down. How in the world do you think you are going to get one?" He smiled knowingly.

After he had left us I thought of the remarkable order, in a sense, that he had constructed out of an essentially chaotic existence, and how his underlying intelligence and charm could have been put to much better use. I also reflected upon the deathly specter that awaits him. JJ had tested positive for HIV (human immunodeficiency virus), although it still lurks within his white cells waiting for something unknown to trigger full-blown AIDS.

JJ did not seem concerned about this, even in the company of the man who shared his room, a demented skeleton, constrained in bed and in the final stages of the disease. JJ will simply go on as he has for as long a time as he has.

JJ has led a life that can only be described as irresponsible and reprehensible, for all his insouciant charm. Yet, as a caring human being and physician, I cannot accept the punishment of AIDS in retribution for it, either for JJ or the many thousands like him.

Once the virus has entered the body it may be as long as ten years before the opportunistic infections or other signs of AIDS will appear in the vast majority of victims. It is in this window of opportunity that I hope and pray that we will come up with some new major effective treatments to combat the disease. Recent combinations of therapeutic agents offer some promise. Whether JJ will be willing or able to avail himself of these remains to be seen. In any event I cannot help rooting for him.

15

A MAN WHAT AM

A SURGEON'S EXIT IN HIGH STYLE

Arnold Armiehalter was a very good man; he just wasn't a very good surgeon. The open heart program he had begun at the hospital was failing and seriously in danger of losing its accreditation. In cardiac surgery, numbers are important. Initial success leads to a growing number of referrals and, inevitably, successful programs prove to be the largest programs. The increasing numbers of patients seem to grease the machine. Whether Arnie's failing program was the result of poor technique or initially poor luck was debatable. What was indisputable was that, just as success builds upon success, failure seems to engender more of the same.

Any surgical program is built around its leader, and as Arnie's early failures impressed themselves upon the members of the hospital staff, the referrals dropped off precipitously. The program was going nowhere, except perhaps to oblivion, and the administration of the hospital, fearful of losing its sizable investment in the facilities provided for this effort, was looking for new leadership. Not only would this bolster the hospital financially—successful open heart programs are big money makers—but the prestige of the institution would be enhanced as well.

Through all this Arnie remained unperturbed and perpetually hopeful. It seemed that it was simply in his nature to be upbeat throughout his life. After enjoying some celebrity as a high school athlete, he attended Annapolis, where he first went out for football. In his mind's eye he could savor in advance his glory day in gridiron history. It is a raw fall afternoon and another classic confrontation is taking place between the rival military academies. The Midshipmen are slightly ahead but, in the last minutes of the game, the West Pointers are on the verge of making the winning touchdown. Suddenly a shattering announcement is heard over the loudspeaker system, electrifying the stands: "Armiehalter in for Navy," as he runs out on the field to save the day. This was not to be; Arnie was just too small and slight for football. He did, however, become a sprinter on the track team, and despite his small stature, his agility and intelligence made him a key playmaker on the basketball team, fueling an enthusiasm for this sport that lasted for the rest of his life. His skillful footwork was repeatedly demonstrated at the hospital staff dinner dances where he wore out one partner after another up to the conclusion of the evening each year.

His other great enthusiasm, after sports, was jazz, and a lifetime of record collecting gave him daily access to everything from early Armstrong through Thelonius Monk. His conversation was peppered with allusions to jazz in his own personalized version of jive talk. When something struck him as particularly fine or memorable, he would beam, "Man, it was what AM," or, more simply, "It was AM!"

Following World War II, Arnie entered medical school under Navy sponsorship and then fulfilled his service obligation in a number of naval hospitals, where his interest in vascular and then cardiac surgery was kindled. Upon discharge from the service, he underwent further surgical training in cardiac procedures and arrived at our hospital full of ideas and the energy to pursue them. It was a good time for newly emerging heart surgeons since the specialty was in its infancy and many hospitals wanted to "get on board" with this promising new field, given the large backlog of patients in need of such treatment.

Not all these programs succeeded, and Arnie's was destined to be one of them. The blow finally fell when the hospital board informed him that he was being removed as head of the heart surgery program. It could not have come as a surprise to Arnie, who was as much a realist as an enthusiast, but it came at a particularly bad time for him. In addition to his failing practice he was experiencing a failing marriage, one which had become loveless as well as childless. His wife was leaving him.

What was he to do with the rest of his life? The performance of surgery has been described as "an athletic event," and, like most tennis players in their thirties, Arnie, a surgeon in his sixties, was past his prime. It was at this point that he turned to a completely different field of endeavor. A local high school, a private institution that did not have to abide by official state requirements for teaching credentials among its staff, was desperately in need of a new athletic director. Arnie, whose passion for sports had never abated, applied for the position and won it.

In the blink of an eye, he resigned his hospital staff position and embarked on a totally new career, one for which he might well have always been better suited. It was not as an athletics director, however, that Arnie distinguished himself, although he performed these duties efficiently. It was in the somewhat related field of officiating at basketball games, first locally and then throughout the county and state, that he began to shine. It was in this role that he finally was achieving the recognition and approval that had eluded him as a physician and surgeon.

I am not a basketball fan; it seems like a pretty pointless exercise to me, throwing balls through baskets. However, spurred on by my earlier friendship with Arnie and glowing reports of his prowess on the court as a referee, I decided to attend one of the games at which he was officiating. As I expected, the game itself was not particularly engrossing; what was infinitely more rewarding was Arnie's display of artistry in his unique but unmistakable way of controlling the game. To call a double dribble, his loud whistle was accompanied by a furious beating of both hands upon imaginary tom-toms. To call charging, he would metamorphose into a locomotive; for blocking, he became a traffic barrier; a traveling call would transform him into a Baryshnikov in slow motion. It was a truly balletic performance.

After the game I congratulated Arnie on his newly found

acclaim, one that he obviously enjoyed as much as his audience. I continued to hear good things about him as one season followed another. We continued to meet for lunch or dinner on occasion, bringing each other up to date on our now totally different professional lives. About three years after his transformation into a local sports celebrity, he experienced an episode of weakness and light-headedness as he left the gym floor. Given his age, it was thought that perhaps this might be the harbinger of a heart condition or even a transient ischemic cerebral attack. He went to a colleague of mine, an internist, for a work-up. It was worse than either. A chest X-ray revealed that his skeleton was riddled with metastatic cancer. His symptoms may well have been related to rising levels of calcium entering his bloodstream from the disintegrating bone, or perhaps as the result of some abnormal hormone being produced by the tumors.

We never found the source of these metastases, the primary tumor, and the disease was not responsive to either chemotherapy or radiation. When his internist asked him about family to consult regarding his condition, Arnie simply mentioned me, and the three of us sat down to discuss the future. Despite the seriousness of the disease and its widespread nature, Arnie suffered little pain, or at least he complained of none, and there were no other disabling symptoms other than occasional episodes of weakness and light-headedness. Although we recognized that death might come at any time, medication could help keep his calcium levels under control and reduce any physical discomfort that might occur. Arnie told us that he intended to carry on as long as he could, and insisted that we keep the knowledge of his condition strictly among the three of us.

Not long after this, one night, after Arnie had exited the basketball court, he was found slumped over lifeless in the locker room. Throughout it all he had remained eternally positive in attitude and uncomplaining. At the funeral, I was asked to give the eulogy. My first inclination, in deference to his courage during those last days, was to pull out that old chestnut about nothing so becoming his life as the manner of his leaving it. But then I thought of how Arnie would have preferred me to express such feelings: He was a man what AM!

16

OTHER FACES OF AIDS

NEW REALITIES TO BE FACED
A QUARTER OF A CENTURY LATER

An infectious disease specialist recently told me, "Almost no one need die from AIDS anymore." Perhaps he should have added "in the United States." The disease that emerged as GRIDS (Gay-related Immunodeficiency Syndrome) in this country in the early 1980s was soon recognized as having extended its domain to involve additional groups. For a time we called them the four H's (adding heroin addicts, hemophiliacs, and Haitians to homosexuals). Now we have come to know that this new disease is no respecter of gender, ethnicity, or nationality. We have learned how it is spread, and we now have a number of drugs at hand that we know can hold it in check if not eliminate it from the body. We are trying to develop a vaccine that may serve to protect the general population as well as those segments most at risk.

Despite the problems still facing health experts in dealing with the AIDS problem, we have come a long way from the era when the diagnosis of AIDS was an absolute death sentence and all victims of the disease could do was to work out painful and sometimes even ingenious ways to cushion their remaining days as best they could. One ploy involved bartering their life insurance policies with grisly entrepreneurs, the patient hoping to obtain financial support during the final days when normal sources of income had dried up, the speculator gambling that the terminal period might not be too prolonged so that any profit might be reduced. One gay acquaintance of mine, luckily having escaped the disease himself, informed me that during this dismal period about 80 percent of his friends—his functioning family in a sense—had succumbed to the disease.

Until fairly recently, as a matter of fact, in this country AIDS was considered as primarily an affliction of gay men by many in the general public. We now know that, worldwide, gay men constitute no more than half of 1 percent of those who contract the disease. Meanwhile, in the United States not only male homosexuals but also intravenous drug addicts, hemophiliacs, and those acquiring the disease through heterosexual contact or at birth (the infants of affected mothers) are virtually guaranteed by federal and state agencies access to medications that will prevent or delay the onset of full-blown AIDS.

But what about the rest of the world where AIDS is spreading unchecked? By the end of 2000 there were already 36.1 million people with HIV/AIDS throughout the world. In 2001 infection with the human immunodeficiency virus (HIV), the cause of AIDS, doubled in Eastern Europe and Central Asia, according to United Nations reports. Neither in these areas nor in Africa, where the disease has already exacted a terrible toll, can this kind of medical care be afforded. In such places the diagnosis of AIDS still carries with it the sentence of death. Efforts to address this problem to date have not been promising. The annual cost of sustaining the life of an AIDS patient in the United States will run from fifteen thousand dollars to more than thirty thousand, depending on the individual case. Even if the cost of instituting such treatment were reduced to one-tenth of this in impoverished areas such as Africa, that sum would still represent significantly more than the total annual income of many of these people.

The danger exists that while we in the United States have come to "live with AIDS," this coexistence might only represent a temporary respite from the disease if the ability of the virus to do us damage outruns our ability to come up with new and effective treatments. Although a number of laboratories have concentrated on developing a vaccine against HIV, such efforts are continually being stymied by the ability of the virus to evade these vaccines. This is because HIV is proving notoriously adept at changing its structure through mutation so that each new formulation of a vaccine developed against an earlier strain of the virus encounters a differently composed and impervious strain when the vaccine is finally administered. This same talent for self-transformation has also resulted in growing resistance to some of the drugs that have held the virus in check in the recent past. Ironically, patients who have been the most reliable and faithful in adhering to such drug regimens are often among those most prone to be found harboring drug-resistant strains of the virus.

Perhaps prevention through health education might prove the most effective way to get the disease under control internationally, but such efforts certainly are not enhanced by governmental leaders such as President Mbeki of South Africa voicing doubts about the nature of the disease, and national leaders elsewhere either denying the existence of the disease in their countries or dragging their feet in addressing the problem, as has often been the case in the past.

Given such ominous portents for the future, it is not beyond the realm of possibility that, despite all the progress we have made, the day may come again when even here in the United States there might be some reversion to the previous state of affairs that once existed in regard to this dreaded disease and continues to be the clinical pattern of the disease in less fortunate countries. What this might mean to future Americans confronting the epidemic can best be characterized by describing some typical experiences of the author with the disease not too long ago when there were minimal pharmaceutical resources to help us in managing it.

Patient 1

M., a twenty-three-year-old man, appeared in our emergency room complaining of some breathlessness and chest discomfort. He certainly did not appear ill at first glance. A splendid specimen of young manhood, he stood at well over six feet in height, an almost exact replica of former baseball idol Darryl Strawberry. But, in addition to his subjective complaints, there were objective findings indicating that there was trouble within.

The veins in his neck were abnormally distended. There was a scratchy to-and-fro sound when the emergency room physician listened to his chest with his stethoscope over the area of the heart, and on the X-ray of the chest the cardiac silhouette was definitely enlarged. An echocardiogram indicated that the enlargement seen on the X-ray film was due to a large amount of fluid in the pericardium, the sac that surrounds the heart. This clinched the diagnosis of pericarditis with a massive amount of fluid compressing the heart, preventing its ability to fill and causing a backup of blood in the veins draining into it: cardiac tamponade.

A pericardiocentesis, placing a small drainage tube into the pericardial space via a needle inserted through the chest wall, was promptly performed to relieve the compression and, following the removal of nearly three liters of bloody fluid, the signs and symptoms of the disorder were relieved—for the moment.

What had caused this to occur in a previously healthy young person? Currently, with all the kidney failure patients on dialysis programs, uremic pericarditis tends to be the most common cause of pericardial effusions of this type. Cancers of the lung or breast might invade the pericardium and result in a similar picture. Tuberculosis was also a possibility, followed by a long list of other less common causes. None of these seemed likely in this case. The most probable cause was one of the ubiquitous common viruses in the environment, usually well tolerated but capable of causing such mischief—viral pericarditis, a condition that is usually self-resolving although often helped along by anti-inflammatory drug treatment. We were about to discover that it was indeed a virus that was the culprit; it was rapidly becoming as ubiquitous as its cousins, but, unlike these other viruses, once settled within the human body, it would in time become anything but tolerable.

At first M. did well. He received some anti-inflammatory drugs by mouth and a small amount had been injected into the pericardial space via catheter at the time the fluid was removed. The pain left, and the fluid did not seem to recur over a two-week period, after which he was discharged from hospital.

Two months later he returned with the same symptoms, but now when the echocardiographic examination was repeated, the ultrasonic picture was different. Within the pericardial space, instead of fluid the predominant substance seemed to be a solid material, suggesting that prominent scar formation was taking place and that this material was now causing the problem: chronic constrictive pericarditis. This can be treated only surgically, and the sooner the better, the scar becoming more adherent to the heart and difficult to remove with the passage of time.

We discussed the problem with our chest surgeons, and we all agreed that removal of the pericardium and the associated scar tissue was the best course to follow. The morning of surgery I was rounding on the medical ward when I received a slightly frantic call from my surgical colleague in the operating room. Upon exposing the contents within the pericardium, he had found something totally unexpected. The tissue that greeted him was not scar but, rather, a gelatinous-appearing bloody red friable mass that bled profusely and involved not only the heart and pericardium but also the adjacent lung.

Following multiple blood transfusions, gingerly placed sutures, and hemostatic packing, the surgeon was able to stem the blood flow and close the chest successfully. The tissue sample sent to the pathology laboratory was diagnosed as an angiosarcoma: Kaposi's sarcoma. At this point, a few more pertinent questions were put to the patient.

It turned out that M. was not homosexual and had never injected drugs either into his veins or under the skin. However, like a number of ambitious youths from the inner city, he had decided that his fame and fortune lay in what was almost becoming a time-honored profession in these places of desperate poverty. He had decided to become a dealer in illicit drugs. Many of his clients turned out to be prostitutes from whom the virile young man often accepted sexual favors in lieu of cash. It was in this way that he had obviously contracted the AIDS virus.

He was placed alone in a room to receive whatever ameliorating medications we could provide. They helped little. He continued to gasp for breath as the flesh melted off that still substantial frame. I stopped by occasionally to offer whatever comfort or encouragement I could. His replies were short, grew shorter, and then became nonexistent. The tumor had entered his brain, and he was in coma. Three months following his second hospital admission he was dead.

PATIENT 2

J. was brought to the hospital by the police. This forty-two-year-old man had been known to be HIV positive for more than three years and already had had several bouts of a lung infection with an opportunistic organism, Pneumocystis carinii (pneumocystis pneumonia or PCP), as well as hepatitis, syphilis, and tuberculosis. He was also a chronic alcoholic and had severe hypertension.

Following an earlier admission for pneumonia he had been

placed on the drug Bactrim, to which PCP often responds, at least at first. However, he became allergic to the drug and it had to be discontinued. He was returned to prison where, for reasons not clear, the Bactrim was resumed. The result was an even more severe allergic reaction involving the skin of his body with blisterlike eruptions, the process also extending to the mucous membranes of his mouth, rectum, and eyes. This constellation of allergic symptoms clearly fell under the heading of Stevens-Johnson Syndrome, one of the few diseases of primarily the skin that can prove fatal if not treated promptly and aggressively.

The patient was placed in isolation and started on massive doses of steroids for the allergic reaction, with antibiotics also given to combat any infection. Local treatment for his skin lesions was also applied. When I first visited his bedside the window shades were drawn and the lights turned down because of his extreme sensitivity to bright light.

A coal-black man, he seemed to blend into the darkness surrounding him, only the whites of his eyes distinctly attesting to his presence. The sores within his mouth prevented him from uttering anything but low, painful moans. Some of the lesions on his torso had broken down, and blood-tinged fluid dripped from his eyes and the sides of his mouth onto his face. He could not unbend his arms or legs because of the painful ulcerations in the skin folds. His whole body gave the appearance of one gigantic, excruciating boil. Even for a seasoned physician the sight was horrifying, and immediately after leaving his room I murmured to my resident, "Poor bastard."

"Maybe you wouldn't be so sorry for him if you knew what he was in jail for," my resident replied. Knowingly a carrier of the AIDS virus, he had raped a four-year-old girl about six months earlier.

A week later J. was clearly responding to the treatment for his skin disease, but something obviously new was going on in his brain. At this point he was observed by his nurse in the process of eating his own feces.

PATIENT 3

The young woman, A., was thirty-three years of age at the time of her admission to my service. As a teenager she had experimented with intravenous drugs on a few occasions, but quickly decided that this was not for her and had given them up. Not so her live-in boyfriend, for whom intravenous drug addiction became a way of life. Before disappearing from her life for good he had left her on welfare with three children, now ages three, four, and six, to care for. It was he who, in all probability, left her with something else as well, as would later become clear.

In the weeks prior to her hospital admission, A. had noticed increasing shortness of breath, the development of a troubling cough, and high fevers. She was admitted to the hospital with the diagnosis of pneumonia. When the outlines of her heart borders on the chest X-ray began to expand and her neck veins bulged we recognized that as with our first patient, M., we were dealing with something in addition to pneumonia: a large pericardial effusion with cardiac tamponade.

The fluid sample from the pericardial space, obtained by needle aspiration, was cultured, and this time indicated a staphylococcal infection. As with any collection of pus, be it under the skin, in the kidney, liver, or elsewhere, the time-honored procedure of surgical drainage was indicated to help clear up the infection.

I was out of town at the time and, for reasons I could not later determine, no tube was inserted into the pericardial space and brought out through the chest wall to allow for drainage. Due to its location, volume, and relative isolation from the distribution throughout the body of intravenously administered antibiotics, the infection in the pericardial space between the heart and the sac containing it remained untouched by such therapy and was allowed to fester.

The high fevers persisted, and over the next two months a succession of life-threatening complications ensued. The lungs, kidneys, and blood-clotting mechanisms all failed intermittently. There was a massive gastrointestinal hemorrhage. Miraculously, the patient survived all this. But then another, quite unusual complication intervened, one that involved me, as a cardiologist, once again directly in the management of the case.

Somehow the continued pericardial infection had eaten its way into the adjacent heart wall and finally completely penetrated it. Blood from within the heart had gushed out into the pericardial space. The patient would have exsanguinated had not the surrounding walls of the pericardium held fast to contain it, at least temporarily.

We were dealing with a pseudo-aneurysm of the heart's left ventricle. With the ordinary ventricular aneurysm there is first a weakening of the heart wall's muscle, most often due to a coronary artery occlusion in the setting of acute myocardial infarction. There follows a bulging out of this thinned, weakened section in a saclike protrusion—a ventricular aneurysm. Occasionally, in such patients, the damaged wall actually ruptures and results in sudden death of the patient unless, fortuitously, the surrounding pericardium manages to contain the internal bleed. The pseudo-aneurysm thus formed—the walls of the aneurysm consisting of heart and pericardium rather than completely heart muscle—is only a temporary reprieve from disaster. In due course the pericardium itself ruptures and the patient bleeds out into the chest cavity. Urgent surgery is performed to close off the abnormal communication between the heart and pericardial space before this occurs.

In A.'s case the pseudo-aneurysm had formed from the opposite direction—pericardium to heart—but the need for repair was no less urgent. The chest surgeons were notified and agreed with the diagnosis, but there was only one impediment to their proceeding with the operation. A blood test performed shortly after A.'s hospital admission had revealed that although she had not reached the stage of clinically apparent AIDS, she was infected with the HIV virus. It had probably been transmitted to her by her erstwhile mate.

None of the surgeons I initially approached was willing to risk self-infection during the course of such an extensive procedure, where finger nicks are not unknown to occur. I argued that with proper care this could be avoided. How many surgeons did they know who had been infected by HIV carriers on whom they operated during the period before we even knew HIV existed? None to my knowledge or theirs. And what about *this* patient? She was certainly worth saving! She had not used drugs for years and certainly was not about to start if she survived this hospitalization. She also was responsible for raising three small children. Yes, she was HIV positive, but when did this occur?

HIV patients may go on for years harboring the virus without experiencing the onset of clinical AIDS with its opportunistic infections, body wasting, or rare neoplastic diseases. As far as ten years out from acquiring the virus as many as 30 percent of HIV carriers will still show no outward evidence of AIDS.

We had no good way to pinpoint when A. had become infected, but if she happened to be among that relatively fortunate 30 percent, she might still have a stretch of good years ahead of her before succumbing. (This was before we had effective agents to hold the disease completely in check for extended periods.) With three small children to raise, this was no minor consideration in my mind. And already at that time we were hopeful that within a few years new drugs would be found either to contain or cure the disease.

Such pleas fell on deaf ears until I approached Dr. Jacques Losman, a relative newcomer to the Newark area. A Belgian by birth, he had been a colleague of Christiaan Barnard during the pioneering heart transplantation work in Cape Town. He agreed to perform the surgical repair of the heart wall, which was accomplished successfully.

All of this occurred more than fifteen years ago. For the few years I continued to follow the progress of A., clinical AIDS did not appear. She put on weight, regained her strength, and was able to attend to the rearing of the three small children in her care. At the time of this writing I still have hopes that this courageous young mother is still as "fat and sassy" as at the time I knew her, and that she is continuing to fulfill her motherhood role thanks to current medications available for the control of AIDS in this country.

I have selected these three cases as a reminder of what AIDS has meant to the American public in the past and what it still represents for millions of less fortunate patients in parts of the world where effective modern treatment is not available. We have heard much of late about the globalization of economies. If this is truly to benefit mankind, it must be realized that inextricably entwined with the economic arm of globalization is its health counterpart. Both must be addressed if the globalization effort is to be truly successful in enhancing the lives of peoples throughout the world.

AIDS is a dirty, desperate business. It will take every resource we have—financial, political, scientific—to deal with it not only with a heightened sense of urgency, but one of reality as well.

17

ON DYING WITH DIGNITY
—AND A DIAGNOSIS

OBJECT LESSONS ON HOW WE CAN NEVER KNOW TOO
MUCH ABOUT PATIENTS AND THEIR ILLNESSES

We have reached a watershed in our thinking about the possibilities and limitations of science. In medicine, particularly, the frequent futility of the mechanistic approach has become widely recognized, and we are beginning to think more about how one might leave this life gracefully and quietly than about new methods of keeping one or another organ system responsive to whatever computerized gadgetry we can devise for the purpose.

In one of the medical periodicals that arrives in our office the issue was stated succinctly in a four-panel cartoon that required no titles other than indications of the day of illness at the top of each. In the left upper panel was drawn the figure of a man in a hospital bed. A tracheostomy tube has been inserted in his neck, and his breathing is being controlled by the respirator to which it is connected. An artificial cardiac pacemaker controls the heartbeat, as indicated on the oscilloscope screen above the bed. Around the bed are hung a string of bottles with various solutions that are being poured into his veins. There are other mechanical support devices (kidney dialysis machine? circulatory assistance device?) in place beside the bed. The panel is labeled "Day 1."

The upper right panel contains a drawing of the same man, identical in every way except for the absence of all the life-support equipment and intravenous lines. It too is labeled "Day 1." The lower left panel represents "Day 11" in the hospital course of the man who has received all the advanced therapy the equipment surrounding him represents. He is draped from head to foot in preparation for his transportation to the morgue. The lower right panel represents the final outcome for the patient who has not received the benefit of advanced medical science. He too has died and is on his way to the morgue. The sign above the illustration reads "Day 10." The dubious benefits of all that advanced medical science are all too apparent.

We have no doubt allowed ourselves to become victimized by our uncritical reliance on the medical machine, and the reaction is setting in. Through the media some years ago we learned of an early decision of one public figure to let nature take its course. Senator Wayne Morse of Oregon, a leader in the upper house for many years, decided to reject the use of a dialysis machine when he learned at an advanced age that he had kidney failure. Another public figure, Charles A. Lindbergh, took a similar stand following his losing battle with cancer as he looked forward to his own last days. Rather than perish in a hospital bed on a cancer service, he chose to fly home to Hawaii and spend his remaining days in the company of his family in the surroundings he loved the most. Several books on the subject of how we should adjust ourselves to the approach of death have become classics on the subject and uniformly stress the need for us to approach the end rationally and in full control.

With all the publicity given the subject of dying, one might infer that this approach is something novel. On the contrary, before the arrival of the electronic age to the bedside, the management of the dying patient was an important component to our medical training. As an intern more than forty years ago, I had a month's rotation on a very special service initiated by Mount Zion Hospital in San Francisco. We young doctors in training were supplied with a battered Plymouth and a list of names, addresses, and charts of patients with chronic illnesses who had elected to receive treatment at home rather than the hospital if at all possible. A number of these were terminal cancer patients whose final days, I believe, were enriched by the presence of family and friends in home surroundings. The adjustment of the families to the deaths of their loved ones was also facilitated by their ability to contribute personally to the care and comfort of the patients during these final days.

The danger now is that the pendulum might have swung too

far. In our striving toward the humanistic approach we must re-member not to fail to cover all avenues of investigation to arrive at the most complete and accurate of diagnoses. We must not fail in our responsibility to explore all therapeutic possibilities that might reasonably offer some chance of success. Three cases come to mind that demonstrate the fineness of the line that physicians must tread in this regard, and suggest the difficulty in establishing future guidelines for the most ethical courses to follow.

CASE I

Mr. Harris was obnoxious. He had little money; he was alone in the world; he was spending his remaining days within a Veterans Hospital; he had incurable cancer; and he was obnox-ious.

He belonged to a species of individuals that are well known to VA hospitals throughout the country. He had served briefly in World War II and had received a minor injury for which he received a disproportionately large disability payment. He had never quite succeeded in civilian society and for most of his post-army life drifted from one menial job to another, often re-quiring some sort of governmental assistance to supplement his meager income. When it was discovered that he had a lym-phoma, a slowly progressive form of blood cancer, he entered a VA hospital for the duration.

This was not a medical necessity. Most civilian patients with this form of cancer might make periodic visits to the hospital for specialized treatment or diagnostic procedures, but in the main they have no difficulty for many years in leading a rela-tively normal existence outside of the hospital until the final stages of the disease, which can be perhaps as many as twenty years following the initial diagnosis. In Mr. Harris's case, however, the massive acquiescence of the VA hospital system made it relatively routine for them to accept him as a permanent resident.

Since Mr. Harris's therapy was intermittent and he was far from bedridden, his days were occupied primarily in nonmedical pursuits within the VA hospital microcosm. He made his daily visits to the coffee shop, the canteen, and the library. He played cards. He played bingo. He watched television. His primary source of recreation, however, it seemed to us on the staff, was baiting the house physician unfortunate enough to have Mr. Harris on his roster of patients and thereby incur the routine of abusive complaints that characterized each morning's rounds.

Undeniably it gave Mr. Harris satisfaction to opine daily that the food was unpalatable, the weather unpleasant, the company disagreeable, and the treatments ineffective. The latter, especially, was an unwelcome barb considering the chronicity of his disease and the fact that his tumors (lymph node swellings) responded so well in shrinking following chemotherapy or X-radiation and that his weight was maintained at near normal throughout his stay, a generally good indication of his overall state of health.

He had been hospitalized for several years by the time I had been assigned to him. I had been warned about the intractability of his disposition, if not his disease, but accepted his multiplicity of complaints as part of the routine in dealing with him. Shortly after my arrival on his ward, however, there was some cause for concern. One of his periodic chest X-rays demonstrated some shadows that were not there before. The radiologist interpreted them as a spread of his lymphoma into the lungs, but the possibility of an infection (pneumonia) was also entertained. Yet, although the latter remained a serious consideration, there was little indication of a pulmonary infection. He had no fever, his blood counts were normal, and the several sputum cultures we obtained showed only the bacteria common to all our mouth cavities ("normal oral flora"). Outwardly, in terms of his general status, he seemed as ornery and combative as ever.

For more than a week we pondered about the diagnosis as we continued to follow his status and examine blood and sputum specimens. It took that long for Mr. Harris to make the diagnosis for us. He did this by dying quite suddenly. At postmortem examination he was found to have a severe pneumonic process involving both lungs. In retrospect we realized that his age and debilitating illness accounted for his body failing to respond to an infection with the fever and other symptoms we might otherwise have expected to find. The medication he received for his cancer had no doubt depressed the bone marrow, preventing the normal rise in white blood cell counts common to bacterial infections. As for the type of bacteria causing the pneumonia, it was the normal oral flora after all that had invaded his lung tissue and were responsible for his demise. Ordinarily unable to cause infections in healthy people because of their low pathogenic potential, these bacteria were able to establish an infection under the conditions that happened to exist in our patient. We realized all this too late to do Mr. Harris any good.

CASE 2

Mrs. Wheeler was the complete antithesis of Mr. Harris. Only in her early fifties, she was a young grandmother who also happened to be vivacious and distinctly glamorous. She was of a distinguished family and had married into an equally highly placed one. Rich and privileged, she nonetheless devoted herself to many public charities as well as private interests. Her many activities were interrupted by a gradually progressive weakness and malaise. She grew pale and depressed. She lost her appetite, and her weight fell. She was admitted to the hospital for evaluation.

An initial series of blood tests revealed that she was in uremia. It was then discovered that both ureters, the tubes leading from the kidneys to the bladder, were blocked off in the lower pelvis. It was the backup of urine through the ureters into the kidneys that was causing the high levels of waste products in her blood stream.

A gynecologist performed a vaginal examination and determined that it was "a frozen pelvis." In other words, he felt that a cancer of the uterus had extended beyond its walls and surrounded the ureters, blocking them off and causing the syndrome that had brought her to medical attention. It was felt to be an untreatable situation, given the therapy available to physicians at that time.

Because of the hopelessness of the prognosis and the relative ease of death from uremia compared with what might be expected in case of a painful spread of the cancer to bony structures, the lungs, and elsewhere, it was decided to allow the uremic process to end her life rather than instituting surgical ureteral bypass procedures that would only be palliative and prolong her life for a limited time.

After Mrs. Wheeler's death several weeks later, a postmortem examination revealed no evidence of uterine cancer or any other. There was, rather, a fibrotic reaction of the connective tissue behind the uterus, and it was this scarring process that involved the ureters, blocking the passage of urine through them. Further investigation revealed that the lady had for some time been subject to migraine headaches and was taking a then new type of medication, methysergide, for this disorder. It was only then that physicians were beginning to recognize retroperitoneal fibrosis as a side effect of the drug; a side effect that could be reversed either by cessation of the drug or surgical means. Had a biopsy been obtained to confirm the clinical diagnosis of "frozen pelvis" and shown that there was no evidence of cancer in the uterus, the diagnosis of the real cause of the uremia might have been discovered in time to save the patient's life.

CASE 3

In the case of Mr. Harris the correct and correctable diagnosis was missed, but not for lack of a conscientious attempt to reach it despite the deceptive clinical setting and the circumstances surrounding it. Despite the patient's resistance to the ministrations of his doctors, despite the complaints and discomforts that might have tended to put one off, despite the lack of cooperation, the bloods were drawn, the sputum collected, the X-rays taken and repeated as they should have been—but all to no avail.

In the tragic case of Mrs. Wheeler, on the other hand, it was an excessive concern for her sensibilities and comfort that clouded the minds of her doctors and precluded the proper performance of their duty.

The final member of this troika of medical dilemmas fortunately provides a happy ending to balance the other two. It was recounted to me by Dr. Samuel A. Levine, a Harvard-based Boston cardiologist who was a contemporary and friend of Paul Dudley White. Although not nearly as well known to the general public as Dr. White, whose far-ranging activities included the care of the ailing President Eisenhower, Dr. Levine was held in equally high esteem for his many accomplishments by all members of the medical profession.

He had been called as a consultant for an opinion regarding the cause of "heart failure" in a seventy-one-year-old dowager. She had been in excellent health throughout her life and had no previous history or symptoms related to heart disease until several months prior to this hospitalization, when her abdomen began to fill with fluid (ascites) and her legs began to swell with edema fluid thought to be secondary to congestion of her veins accompanying heart failure. Her family physician had thought that in a woman of her advanced years the most likely cause was arteriosclerotic heart disease (what we would now call coronary heart disease) and that symptomatic treatment of the fluid accumulation by the limited number of medications available for this purpose was all that could be offered until death claimed her.

Dr. Levine was troubled by the diagnosis of the case. With no previous episodes of heart pain (angina pectoris) and no evidence of heart damage on the electrocardiogram of disease that might have otherwise gone unnoticed by the patient, he was reluctant to accept the diagnosis of arteriosclerotic heart disease, despite the relatively advanced age of the patient. As for an alternate possibility of valvular heart disease causing heart failure, the typical murmurs indicating this were absent. There were, however, some features to suggest another possibility. This was constrictive pericarditis, chronic inflammation and scarring of the sac around the heart, which could prevent the heart chambers from filling adequately and in turn cause a backing up of the blood returning to the heart with all the features of venous congestion also seen in chronic heart failure resulting from intrinsic disease of the heart itself.

The significance of entertaining this diagnosis was that it would involve a radical course of action for that time. The chest would have to be opened for surgical exploration to determine if this was indeed the case, and whether removal of the pericardium might be accomplished. This problem had presented itself to Dr. Levine and his colleagues long before such specialized procedures of cardiac catheterization and cardiac angiography had been introduced. And, parenthetically, even today with these procedures available along with CT scanning and magnetic resonance imaging, the diagnosis is often a difficult one to establish without surgical exploration.

At that time not only was diagnosis difficult but also direct heart surgery itself was scarcely in its infancy, and open heart surgery had yet to be performed. If this elderly sick lady was placed under general anesthesia and her chest opened only to find that constrictive pericarditis was not the cause of her symptoms, with severe heart disease present she might not survive even an exploratory operation. Was this a risk worth taking? In Dr. Levine's opinion it was.

Even with excellent management of the symptoms related to congestion of the vascular system, it would only be a holding action. On the other hand, if constrictive pericarditis was the cause of the patient's illness, removal or "stripping" of the pericardium from the surface of the heart chambers would enable them to fill and empty in a normal manner once more. The situation was discussed with the elderly lady, who decided to have them proceed with the operation.

After much nay-saying and head-wagging on the part of others, Dr. Levine's opinion prevailed. The surgery was performed, constrictive pericarditis was indeed discovered, the pericardium was stripped, and the patient sailed through the operation with no complications and in the weeks succeeding completely rid herself of all the fluid that had accumulated over the past months—with no medication whatsoever. How much was gained?

The scene changes to a European capital twelve years later where Dr. Levine is attending an international heart disease symposium as a guest lecturer. As he pauses on one of the boulevards, he feels a hand on his arm. He turns to see before him that same "invalid" who, in her eighty-third year, is in the process of taking a world tour. She had learned their paths were crossing in this particular city and simply wished to greet him and thank him again before rushing to complete a life still full of substance and adventure.

Some might argue that given the current advanced status of medical technology, diagnoses such as those missed in our first two patients and made only with great difficulty in the third would now be made with ease routinely, that misdiagnosis of patients is now a rare occurrence. Such thinking certainly dominates much of the medical community as well where autopsies, at least in the United States, have fallen to a historical low.

However, a recent autopsy study evaluating our modern physicians' ability to make precise diagnoses indicates something different. It demonstrated that even in a university hospital setting where the best brand of medicine might be expected to flourish, in 10 percent of the patients autopsied a major diagnosis was missed which, had it been recognized and treated, would have prolonged the life of the patient. In an even greater number of instances there were minor diagnoses missed that, although not life-threatening, might have eased the clinical course of the patients if diagnosed and managed properly.

Such data should be humbling to all of us in the profession and serve as a caution to us and our patients. We should recognize that even with all the technical paraphernalia at our disposal, we can still miss important illnesses. Together, with our patients' understanding and cooperation, we should resolve to leave no stone unturned to find and treat the causes of their distress before allowing them to simply die undiagnosed in dignity.

18

THE GIFT

WHAT "A GOOD DOCTOR" REALLY MEANS

What, I kept wondering, were those cartons of partially un-wrapped stereo components doing in the middle of the living-room floor in my friend's vacation cottage out on Cape Cod? It was especially puzzling because the year before he had already installed similar equipment to enjoy during his family's sum-mer holidays. My friend Sandy, a classmate from many years back in medical school, proceeded to explain.

Some weeks earlier, late on a Friday afternoon as he was about to leave on vacation from his office in a suburban New York community, he was visited by an old patient who had ca-sually dropped by to discuss what he believed to be a minor problem. About a month previously he had begun to experi-ence some pain in his left hip. The pain was not severe or pro-gressive, but it was persistent and had led the patient, fairly savvy in the ways of the medical world, first to seek out the help of a neurologist and then an orthopedic surgeon before calling on Sandy.

Neither of the other physicians had come up with a satisfying answer to the complaint. The orthopod had, however, taken X-ray films of the hips and pelvis. The only positive finding was a "bone island," an area of increased density that was not in the location of the complaint and carried with it no particular pathological significance. He nonetheless thought it might be a good idea for the patient to undergo an additional study, a bone scan, that might shed some light on whatever was the source of the trouble. The patient had elected to see Sandy, his personal physician, to follow up on this suggestion.

Sandy is a cardiologist who now limits his practice to that subspecialty. However, like all subspecialists in internal medi-cine, he had first become certified in the broader area of general medicine, and early in his career, before he had found it possi-ble to practice cardiology exclusively, he took on a number of patients for general medical care to help pay the bills. Many of these finally left for one reason or another, but a few old faithfuls had remained with him through the years. One of these was this patient, Steve, a successful attorney in his late forties.

A bone scan is a relatively routine procedure. A small amount of radioactive material is injected intravenously and then the whole body is scanned to detect its distribution. Any areas of increased uptake are called "hot spots" and may indicate a variety of abnormal conditions including infection, arthritis, other inflammatory conditions, trauma, or, most ominously of all, cancer arising in bone or spread there from other sites within the body. Depending upon the location or patterns of such hot spots, further diagnostic studies may then be undertaken to define the cause more specifically with an eye to appropriate therapy.

Sandy referred Steve for the bone scan to the radiology department of the local hospital, situated just across the street from his group's office building. As an additional precaution he had his nurse draw a blood sample for several screening tests to be performed later that evening and checked on the following Monday. Steve left reassured, but unbeknown to Sandy, he was late on his way to his own vacation home, in Connecticut, for a weekend's relaxation before returning to work the following Monday. He happened to have had business connections with a number of hospitals, including one in rural Connecticut very close to his vacation home. He knew that simply by giving Sandy's name as the referring physician he could have the study performed in this more convenient location.

About ten o'clock Friday evening, when Sandy arrived at his place on the Cape, there were two urgent messages awaiting him. One was from his patient, Steve, and the other from David, a new cardiologist who had just joined Sandy's practice. Sandy sensed a connection and decided that the wiser course would be to call his colleague first to see what was up. David was taking weekend call and, in Sandy's absence, it was he who had received a telephone call from the radiologist in Connecticut who had just examined the results of Steve's bone scan. The radiologist revealed to David that on the scan there were a number of areas of increased uptake found: one was in the region of the left hip, the source of Steve's pain, but there were also two ribs involved as well as one of the vertebrae in the patient's spine. All were "consistent with" metastatic cancer or perhaps multiple myeloma, a type of blood cancer primarily residing in the bone marrow and characteristically causing symptoms of bone pain to those afflicted with it.

Following the bone scan, the demeanor of the radiologist no doubt alerted Steve to some potentially important problem. Although no details were given to the patient, he was advised to consult his private doctor about it. Steve had called David in Sandy's absence and the new associate, who knew nothing prior about this particular patient, simply gave an evasive reply, referring the patient in turn to my friend at the Cape. He hoped he had done the right thing and was assured by Sandy that he had handled it very well.

Sandy was devastated. How could he have missed it? How could he have failed this patient, not only one of long standing but who was also his personal lawyer and friend? He recalled how, after his cardiology practice had been built up sufficiently, he had offered Steve the opportunity to change internists and how Steve had replied. The words echoed in his ears: " I'll stick with you because I trust you more than any doctor I know."

It was the ultimate compliment, especially from one who had so many dealings with hospitals and doctors and was well acquainted with their world. Sandy, in turn, had tried to live up to the trust that had been placed in him. Each year when he gave Steve his annual physical examination he touched every medical base from head to toe. But, in truth, it was the kind of thoroughness that he lavished upon all of his patients. He is that kind of doctor.

How then could he have failed his patient in such an egregious way? As he pondered about what to say when he returned Steve's call, his wife tried to comfort him. Despite the ominous portents of the situation and her husband's obvious distress over them, she, at least, managed to handle it rather well.

"Sandy, don't jump to conclusions. After all a bone scan is only one test, and perhaps there is a much simpler and even harmless cause to what the doctor saw on the bone scan."

My friend, however, could only envision the worst scenarios conceivable. The possibilities of various kinds of cancer immediately came to mind. Steve was a nonsmoker, so a metastatic lung cancer was unlikely. But prostate cancer typically goes to bone, and although on the young side for this particular malignancy, Steve could certainly have harbored one. Frantically, Sandy tried to remember whether or not on that last physical he had felt the prostate adequately on rectal examination. Steve had had some complaints about urinary frequency that might have indicated an enlarged, possibly cancerous, prostate, but Sandy had discounted them. Had he missed a hard nodule of prostate cancer, at that time? Had he requested a PSA (prostatic specific antigen) test in the blood work he had ordered before leaving for vacation? Although it could be a source of confusion in many patients—it is elevated in other prostate conditions besides cancer and there is a wide gray area between normal and clearly abnormal—at this point he felt it was only another item of omission in his deplorable handling of the case. Then multiple myeloma again reared its ugly head in his differential diagnosis, and he was convinced that he certainly had never done anything to explore this as a possibility.

Finally, he got hold of himself adequately enough to call his friend and patient in Connecticut. He spoke about the abnormal bone scan in as calm a manner as he could manage and emphasized that it would be unwise to jump to conclusions. But Steve, who knew Sandy only too well, could easily detect the underlying concern. Despite this, he seemed to be handling the news remarkably well. In fact, Sandy observed inwardly, *everybody* seemed to be handling it pretty well with the exception of himself. They agreed to meet the following Monday morning in Sandy's office, where Steve would bring the films that had been turned over to him by the Connecticut radiologist.

My friend spent a sleepless night wondering what next to do. He did not yet know the results of the blood tests he had ordered before he had left Friday evening, and even if they did not include those about which he was most concerned, he knew his staff always saved a little extra blood sample just in case additional tests were required. But, it being summer, there was another problem: the office was closed on Saturdays, and the doctors were on call only for hospital emergencies. Nevertheless, he was able to take some positive steps. He called the radiology department in Connecticut. The radiologist in question was off duty and not reachable. However, the technician on duty was able to read him the precise words of the report. It was as bad as he originally feared.

He then called his own hospital's radiology department to consult their chief, for whom he had tremendous respect and admiration. Although the radiologist was off duty, he called in for any messages that evening and responded to Sandy's inquiry immediately. He too knew Steve personally and indicated that he would be happy to come in Sunday morning and meet with the patient and Sandy to evaluate the situation. Sandy called Steve about this possibility, but Steve had obviously recovered his balance better than Sandy. He calmly indicated it could wait until Monday.

As soon as Sandy arrived in the office Monday morning, he checked the chemistries that he had ordered the previous Friday. Those among them which might have indicated some bone invasion by cancer proved to be normal. A rapid run of the remaining sample for PSA was also unquestionably normal. Sandy began to breathe a little easier.

A call then came from his radiologist, to whom Steve had come directly with the bone scan films. Although there were definite abnormalities, he reported, there was nothing on the films that he found convincing to point to cancer, at least in the ribs and spine. Several benign conditions were much more likely possibilities. As for the hip, however, he felt that, as a further part of the work-up, an MRI (magnetic resonance imaging) scan on Steve would be helpful, and Sandy concurred.

Later that day a more definite conclusion would be reached. The MRI exam convinced the radiologist that the problem in the left hip was a rare condition called transient osteoporosis. Although regular X-rays of the hip joint are normal early in the course of the disorder, as was the case with Steve, The MRI shows characteristic early abnormalities. Later the hip will show bone loss or osteoporosis on the standard film, but this will almost invariably resolve with simple conservative treatment. Over the next few weeks, as predicted, this is precisely what occurred.

As for the other hot spots revealed on the bone scan, nothing further developed to indicate that they represented anything of a serious, potentially lethal nature. Multiple myeloma was soon ruled out by specific blood testing performed for this purpose, and the crisis was over.

Ever so often some tabloid will publish a list of The Best Doctors you can find in your community. In my own area I peruse these with some amusement. Some of the doctors chosen are indeed known to me to be superb, but others, whatever their public standing, I know to be wanting in the realm of individual patient care.

I do not doubt that those who compile these lists try to be fair and accurate, but I wonder how they go about it. Do they just look up lists of professors at medical schools and chiefs of departments at prominent hospitals? Do they take a sampling of opinion from doctors in the community? Do they check the Index Medicus for numbers of publications? Maybe they also just ask their friends. But whatever qualities they do seek in a physician to merit such an accolade, there is one which I am sure that they do not consider, and that is the ability to worry.

A doctor can be keenly intelligent, superbly trained, and widely respected by his colleagues, but, for myself, although I would desire these attributes, more than anything else I would seek in a personal physician the irresistible compulsion to worry about me. I really want them to have restless moments and even sleepless nights (when I am really ill) to ensure that I am getting the very best of medical care.

Sandy is not a professor; he is not a chief of any department; he does not publish research papers; I doubt that he has any magazine editors among his patients. However, he happens to be keenly intelligent, very well trained in his profession, and scrupulous about keeping up to date in his field. He is also utterly devoted to his patients. He worries about them constantly. Not only close friends like Steve, but all of them. It takes a toll on him, as it does on other doctors of a similar nature, but that is what makes them such fine practitioners of the art and science of medicine.

After this whole episode had worked itself out to its conclusion, Steve became aware of the distress and anxiety that his physician had endured on his behalf. He felt that he had to send some token of appreciation to demonstrate the esteem in which he held his doctor. So that was the reason for that hi-fi set in the middle of the living room up on the Cape. And as for Sandy—I think he deserved every decibel of it.

19

Time (Overdue) for a Change

Random Insanity:
Examples from the American Health Care System

In any discussion of health care reform, mention is made of America's uninsured population, now approaching fifty million. Here is the story of one of them.

Mrs. C. entered the United States from South America in 1979 at the invitation of her eldest son, who had preceded her into the country some years before. Accompanying her were her three daughters, their husbands, and a growing band of grandchildren. The entire family moved into a large, multibedroom house where Mrs. C. remained to care for the little ones while the other adults went to seek and find employment.

Until 1989 Mrs. C. had the good fortune of maintaining her usual state of robustly good health. Then, at the age of sixty, she became ill. Neither she nor her children had ever been able to afford private health insurance.

First there was a lump in the breast, which turned out to be cancerous. A mastectomy and subsequent follow-up treatments were provided. Three years later she suffered a coronary occlusion and a massive heart attack (myocardial infarction) that led to her hospitalization for several weeks. She emerged from this only a shade of her former self. The following year she noticed some vaginal bleeding and, after being bounced back and forth from one hospital clinic to another, she came to the attention of one of our gynecological surgeons. He felt a pelvic mass and admitted her to the hospital for removal of what he strongly suspected to be uterine cancer.

I was called to give medical clearance for the surgery to be performed and noticed a prominent heart murmur as well as congestive changes in the lungs indicating heart failure. A severely leaking heart valve related to her previous myocardial infarction was the most likely cause. She was also febrile at this time, and blood cultures and ultrasonic examinations of her heart indicated that the valve had become infected (bacterial endocarditis). A six-week course of antibiotics cleared up the infection, and medical treatment considerably relieved the signs and symptoms of heart failure.

However, her cardiac condition still seemed too precarious to risk major abdominal surgery without significant worsening of her heart failure. I suggested that perhaps laparoscopy could be performed. With minor abdominal incisions made to allow visualization of the mass, I felt that biopsies might be obtained to either confirm or deny the surgeon's suspicions. Perhaps the radical surgery he envisioned might be avoided. The surgeon vetoed this suggestion. The odds were overwhelming that the mass was indeed cancerous, and such biopsies would run the risk of seeding the abdominal wall with the tumor cells and thus preclude any curative effects of the surgery. The diseased valve would have to be replaced with an artificial one before the cancer surgery could be performed safely.

A heart catheterization confirmed the previous assessment of her cardiac condition and, importantly, indicated that the valve replacement could be performed without the additional need for coronary bypass surgery at the same time. The valve was replaced successfully, and a month later the diseased uterus along with the tubes and ovaries were removed without incident. The pathological reports indicated this new cancer had almost completely invaded her reproductive organs. Fortunately, it had not spread beyond them, and a course of chemotherapy was undertaken to ensure, hopefully, that a full recovery would be obtained for this now sixty-three-year-old woman.

Although Mrs. C.'s devoted children tried to pay for some of her medical bills at various times during her extended illnesses, the sums involved soon became astronomical. From our hospital alone she received a preliminary bill of more than $150,000, exclusive of physicians' fees. The hospital, obviously following some regulations as well as practical considerations in regard to the bill, never pursued the matter. I and the other physicians involved in the care of the patient provided our services gratis, being fully cognizant of the patient's financial status. The family could not afford to pay; she was ineligible for Medicaid; she was too young for Medicare; and only if she were completely and permanently bedridden or insane would she fit into some program that would meet any part of her financial needs.

During the time I was shepherding Mrs. C. through this maze of medical miracles, my thoughts turned to my barber, Mario. Every few weeks as he trimmed my hair he gave me updates on his own medical problems. Mario was also an immigrant, but his arrival had preceded Mrs. C.'s by many years. Arriving in the United States at the age of twenty-one, the industrious barber from Naples, after working for an older man, was soon able to open his own shop, marry, and raise a family in his own version of living the American dream.

For thirty years he had maintained a family policy with Blue Cross/Blue Shield and, fortunately, rarely needed to rely upon it. Then, in 1988, he was found to have severe coronary disease requiring bypass surgery. Soon thereafter he was required by the insurance company to remove himself from the family policy and begin paying annual additional charges for himself— thousands of dollars he could ill afford. He sought relief from this oppressive cost by switching to another insurance company, where he was led to believe his costs of cardiac care would eventually be covered. He bitterly learned the meaning of "pre-existing condition": it would be two years before coverage for this would kick in under the new policy. During this time other complications of his disease arose but, gritting his teeth, Mario found means to pay for the additional care out of pocket while anxiously awaiting for the two-year period to end and the new policy to pick up all future costs.

Not surprisingly, when the policy came up for renewal two years later, there was nothing to indicate this provision in the fine print. All those prior assurances had disappeared, along with the salesman who had sold him the policy. In Mario's words, "I found a cart with no wheels."

The coronary grafts by this time had probably closed or new obstructions had occurred because Mario was now in heart failure, poorly controlled by multiple medications. By the end of each day at the barber chair his ankles were swollen with fluid and he found himself gasping for breath. He developed a serious irregularity of the heartbeat (atrial fibrillation) for which he was placed on anticoagulation therapy to prevent blood clots from forming within the heart and then possibly breaking off (embolizing) to the brain or elsewhere in the body. Frequent laboratory checks of his blood were required because of difficulty in controlling his blood-clotting at optimal levels. He had a gastrointestinal bleed, possibly from a small ulcer, and required treatment to prevent a recurrence. In addition to his anticoagulant medicine he eventually was taking eleven other medications. His medical costs, amounting to thousands of dollars each year, ate up a third of his total income. He was ineligible for Medicare because he continued to work. If he chose to retire because of his illness and go on total disability this would place him in an even deeper financial hole. Mario was now fifty-four years old, and he would not live to see his fifty-fifth birthday. He died at home.

Some years later my thoughts return to Mrs. C. I marvel at how well she was served by the medical system at that time, despite the fumbling and infuriating bureaucratic hurdles it sometimes entailed. Hers was not an isolated case. Having worked all my professional life at urban medical centers to which the poor invariably turn for care, I can attest that such treatment has traditionally been proffered without a second thought as to cost or ability to pay. In the past the costs of such care have been absorbed by state or municipal governments and the public hospitals that cater to such patients. Mrs. C. was remarkable only in the extent of the care provided. Today, with the increasing financial squeeze to which such institutions are subjected, I doubt if such care could be so readily provided—if it could be provided at all.

What I have begun to wonder about even more are the millions of Americans like Mario who are not yet quite destitute enough to merit charity care. Despite the institution of some reforms in the health insurance industry, many like Mario anguish each day over each new bill, and ration their own care or medications because they do not have the insurance coverage or the ready cash to pay for them. How many other Marios are being victimized by their own commitment to middle-class values such as paying your own way?

The insanity and unfairness of a system that operates in such a manner can no longer be tolerated. Late in 2005 the Comptroller General of the United States estimated that unfunded obligations of big entitlement programs, including Social Security, Medicare, and Medicaid, amounted to a national debt that will amount to forty-two trillion dollars, including the eight-trillion-dollar unfunded liability of a new Medicare drug benefit that no one seems to understand. In recent years we have witnessed the heavy-handed and misguided attempts of the Clinton administration to grapple with health care funding. The current Bush administration has seemed only intent on lining the pockets of the rich at the expense of the poor. The Congress seems incapable of any actions other than supporting the ill-advised tax cuts of the Bush White House and passing pork barrel legislation to an unprecedented amount. Neither branch of government seems capable of addressing the tsunami of financial burden that future health costs will entail.

Single-payer programs have been recommended, and they

seem to offer some hope for the future, although we are becoming aware of how other advanced nations, despite guaranteeing universal "free" health care, are often facing severe financial difficulties of their own. Meanwhile, the United States, which boasts the best modern health care available in the world, is finding that millions and millions more of its citizens are unable to avail themselves of it.

20

STROKE

A FAMILY AFFAIR

December 1977 found Gregory K., at forty-one years of age, nearing the pinnacle of his career as a successful cardiologist. Well-trained, extremely bright, and industrious, he had earned the respect of his colleagues and the admiration of the many patients crowding his office. In terms of personality, Greg was unusually conservative for such a time. Although possessed of a wry sense of humor, which he readily shared with others, his formality in speech and dress set him apart. Assured in manner and elegantly attired in his well-tailored suits, he could best be described as reassuringly magisterial as he appeared in the office setting or on the wards of the hospital.

On this evening, however, Greg had decided to put aside his professional responsibilities for a few hours, signing out to another colleague so that he might attend a special Boy Scout meeting with his son. His wife, Marsha, and the boy's older sister completed the family outing. For a few days prior to this, Greg had been having some headaches, but nothing he interpreted as really out of the ordinary. He thought they were probably just a reflection of the increasing workload of his burgeoning practice.

Midway through the program Greg realized that he had left his beeper on the kitchen table at home, no more than a few minutes away, and that he would have to retrieve it. He told his wife that he would soon rejoin them at the scout meeting. He never did.

When Marsha returned home with the children, she found her husband seated at the kitchen table complaining again of a headache and seeming not quite himself. "Probably just a touch of the flu," he assured her, and they retired to bed. During the night Greg, as he often did, mumbled in his sleep, but this increased toward morning with an increase in the headache as well as he awoke. He began to lose consciousness. This led to an ambulance pick-up and transportation to the emergency room at the local hospital with which Greg was affiliated.

Cerebral angiography was performed soon after. This revealed that Greg had suffered a major brain hemorrhage, although the precise source of this could not be identified. The hemorrhage was associated with increased intracranial pressure. To prevent this from affecting vital brain functions, a neurosurgeon inserted a tube into one of the fluid-containing cavities of the brain with drainage to the abdominal cavity (a ventriculoperitoneal shunt). A tracheostomy was performed to allow for assisted respiration as the patient became even less responsive. Weeks passed as they attempted to stabilize Greg so that he could be transferred to a medical center in New York for further diagnosis and treatment. Before this could be arranged, two more massive bleeds occurred, threatening any future attempts at surgical rescue.

Transfer was, however, successfully achieved after a total of three months at the community hospital. At the university hospital in New York, additional angiographic studies of the circulation to the brain revealed the culprit to be a leaking berry aneurysm, a thin-walled swelling of one of the arteries at the base of the brain often prone to rupture. Greg had already beaten the odds by surviving three major bleeds. Surgical clipping at the neck of the aneurysm was the only way to ensure that a fourth and possibly fatal bleed might not occur. There were additional delays in performing this surgery for a variety of technical reasons while the surgeon awaited the optimal time to intervene. Greg drifted in and out of consciousness.

Providentially, no paralysis had occurred. The aneurysm was located at the base of the brain rather than in the vicinity of areas controlling motor function. The cerebellum, however, was in close proximity to it, and this area of the brain is important for maintaining a sense of balance among other functions. The loss of balance would plague Greg for months and years to come. About two weeks after his admission to the university hospital, successful clipping of the aneurysm was finally accomplished.

During the first months of his confinement at the new hospital, Greg had become resistant to feeding, eventually losing about sixty pounds of weight. At one point a nasogastric tube had to be inserted to ensure adequate food intake. The probable cause for this behavior, not clear at the time but obvious in retrospect, was the onset of a severe depression, undiagnosed until much later after his discharge from this second hospital six months after the onset of his illness.

Throughout the early course of his hospitalization there was concern over the extent to which he might have suffered some cognitive impairment. At the medical center an I.Q. test was administered. His wife was informed that the result of his performance was average. This was not encouraging since Greg had been tested frequently as a child and young man and had achieved very high scores every time. His performance at this stage, I believe, was impaired by the undiagnosed depression. I actually administered my own intelligence test each time I visited him around the time of his surgery. I would arrive with an entirely fictionalized, complicated cardiological case that I claimed to have been baffling me. When I asked Greg for his thoughts on the make-believe patients his analyses were always clear, concise, and right on the mark. There was no doubt in my own mind about the preservation of his mental faculties. Nonetheless, following whatever brief conversations we had he would soon become less communicative. He would often ask me about my own recent activities and the latest gossip at the medical school. I would then begin my monologue, only to have it interrupted by Greg's deep snoring as he lapsed back into semi-consciousness.

While I observed no lack of cordiality to me from my friend, the same sort of treatment was not afforded his family, to whom he became very distant. His wife recalled how her visits to his bedside were barely acknowledged. His illness, about which he obviously felt shame and helplessness, affected his relationship with his children as well. They were asked not to come to the hospital while he was incapacitated, and he did not attempt to contact them by telephone. At one point his thirteen-year-old son accused his mother and grandparents of deceiving him. He thought that his father had died and that their supposed visits to the hospital to see him were a sham to conceal this from him and his sister. Only after Greg was informed of this did he finally call his children and try to reassure them. However, the anger and depression that had engulfed Greg only served to alienate him once and for all from both his children. His daughter, just entering the difficult teenage years at the time of his illness's onset, was remarkably intelligent but as willful as her demanding father. The tug of war between them was only exacerbated by his stroke, and for the remaining years of his life they were never reconciled. His son, a bit younger than his sister, had never established strong bonds with his doctor father up to the time of his stroke, and in the ensuing years, in an estrangement less overt than his sister's, he gradually drifted away from any emotional contact with his father.

While this disruption of normal relationships with his wife and children was taking place, his and Marsha's parents suffered as well. Greg's mother kept a tearful vigil outside his hospital door, constantly berating herself and wondering what it was that she had done wrong to cause her son so terrible a fate. Later on the two sets of elderly grandparents took to accusing each other of inadequate support for the stricken couple and their children.

On the strictly medical front, following the surgery there was a bit of right-sided weakness observed that was thought not to be critically disabling. Some difficulty with balance was of more concern, and there were some minor visual difficulties. Greg had alternated between a walker and cane to help himself to and from the bathroom of his hospital room. The need for rehabilitative therapy was recognized, and Greg was assigned to a physical and occupational therapist.

Right from the beginning there was conflict with this woman, who focused on, of all things, Greg's color blindness, a condition he had had all his life. She insisted it was simply a question of mind over matter and that if Greg would only put his mind to the problem it would no longer be a matter. Even in his debilitated state Greg could not let this absurdity pass. Along with his loss of respect for her knowledge of ophthalmology came his loss of confidence in any other of her abilities. In the eyes of the rehabilitation staff, such impertinences marked him as a troublemaker. It was all downhill from there. He entered the program with a cane and walker; he emerged from it two months later in a wheelchair.

By this time, six months after the start of Greg's illness and three months into his hospitalization at the medical center, the crushing economic realities of his situation were becoming clear to Greg and Marsha. A representative from the hospital, a social worker, called Marsha in for a meeting. The bill at the hospital had now reached $75,000 ($250,000 in today's dollars), and most of it was not covered by their medical insurance. The social worker then asked if, by any chance, Greg had had any military service. She learned that Greg had served in the U.S. Air Force as a flight surgeon during the Vietnam War.

"You're saved," she informed Marsha.

Greg was transferred to a Veterans' Administration hospital near their home where there was an excellent rehabilitation service in operation. Marsha also learned at this time that one could actually negotiate with hospitals for their bills and, in exchange for payment in cash, the university hospital accepted a substantial reduction in the balance of the bill.

Their experience with the community hospital where Greg had been on staff was very different. No bill was ever sent to them for the three months he was confined there. In those days things were different. A loyal and respected attending physician was afforded this kind of generosity when such a medical disaster had suddenly halted his earning capacity. The medical staff responded in kind, taking up a collection for Greg to help him manage during the early days of his illness. The county medical society also chipped in with a small contribution. Some cardiologists on staff filled in on caring for his patients while expressing hopes for his rapid return to practice.

This was not soon in coming. Following his discharge from the VA hospital, Greg spent a year at home recuperating. In 1979 he felt well enough to resume his practice. This was two years from the time of the initial cerebral hemorrhage. Prior to his illness he had been interviewing a number of younger men to join him in his rapidly expanding practice. Now no one seemed interested, nor was there a need for a partner in a practice that had dwindled considerably. He had a feeling of disorientation, what he described as "feeling like a Rip van Winkle coming back after twenty years in the mountains" in a letter to the editor he wrote in response to an article by another physician recounting his own experiences following a serious illness.

It was not easy to resume work. Although Greg found the nurses encouraging and cheerful, such attitudes were not universal at the hospital. "Some of my old friends were very helpful but others carefully avoided me and crossed to the other side of a hallway when they saw me coming and avoided sitting with me in the hospital food shop. Others seemed openly angry that I had the temerity to get better."

Patients also avoided him. Those who are ill and living with serious threats to their physical well-being prefer having a physician who exudes strength and security. The new Dr. K., with a prominent depressed scar on his forehead, clothes hanging loosely on his diminished frame, and hobbling about with the aid of a cane, was no longer either reassuring or magisterial in appearance.

The right-sided weakness, something discounted at first, became more pronounced, making it difficult for Greg to move about. For some years he had suffered from "arthritis" in the neck, which limited his range of head motion in addition to causing pain. Could his weakness be related to disc problems in the neck vertebrae? A myelogram revealed some pathology in this region, and laminectomies of several cervical vertebrae were performed. No improvement was observed post-operatively and the condition continued to progress.

With much courage, Greg tried to erase the image of incapacity that he presented to staff and patients at the hospital. He attempted to carry on without a cane, but suffered several falls due to his loss of balance and weakness. One day after a severe fall in the hospital parking lot he was returned home bleeding profusely from multiple cuts and bruises. All these developments led to his final retirement from active practice in 1987, eight years after his attempted resumption of work. By this time he was seeing only six or eight patients a week, hardly enough to justify maintaining an office. The practice was not offered for sale. There was now no practice to speak of.

As time went on the weakness that he had experienced on the right side extended to the left side of the body as well. He had difficulty keeping his head erect, and one had to adapt an awkward position below his head level to come into Greg's line of vision. No type of ambulation was now possible. Greg had to be transported in a wheelchair. A special hospital bed was installed in the first-floor dining room of the home, which became his world for the remaining fifteen years of his life.

One physical indignity after another was heaped upon him. He became unable to move his bowels and needed to be cleaned out every few days. At one point he became focused on some abdominal swelling that he attributed to retained feces. Finally it became apparent that the bulge in his lower abdomen was not intestine but a bladder distended with several pints of urine as the result of an enlarged prostate. The transurethral prostate-ctomy relieved the obstruction but left him incontinent, requir-ing a condom catheter for the rest of his life.

Although his clinical depression had now been recognized and he was under medication for this, he became subject to anxiety attacks. It was often difficult to distinguish between these and truly physical complaints. Was the breathlessness of which he often complained a reflection of his mental state or evidence that the paralysis that had begun to invade his chest muscles was affecting his respiratory function? He was fitted with a sort of cuirass device to help him breathe more nor-mally, but he could not tolerate it. He rejected any thought of having a tracheostomy performed because of the effect this would have on his failing ability to speak clearly and loud enough to be heard.

As Greg's health declined, so did his family life. As children grow older and enter maturity, their lives naturally deviate from the home environment. But in this household such tendencies were markedly exacerbated as a result of Greg's condition. The daughter in particular, so close to her father before the stroke, could not face the remnants of the once powerful and loving figure to whom she was attached and rarely visited him. Greg's father, who had become a widower since the onset of his son's illness, found himself once again in love in his eighties and re-married. It was almost as if a malevolent power had restored the old man's vitality and zest for life simply to mock the unin-terrupted descent of his son into invalidism.

The one remarkable positive development within this per-sonal tragedy was the emergence of Marsha as a figure of unimag-ined strength, resourcefulness, and determination. Small and frail in appearance, she had often seemed to friends immature and even flighty before her husband's illness. This wisp of a woman was the last person in the world one would have be-lieved capable of becoming the rock upon which her family clung for so many years. A sheltered only child and pampered to excess by her doting parents, she had no professional training and seemed destined only for the dependent role of wife to a powerful and protective spouse such as Greg once was. Indeed, she believed that it was her very vulnerability that attracted Greg to her in the first place. He gloried in being her protector and provider.

She learned how to deal with hospital functionaries, lawyers, and creditors. She learned how to stretch dollars well beyond their prescribed limit. She had to. Although Greg had purchased total disability insurance prior to his stroke, they learned that such policies were often best suited to men in their sixties with the expectation of only a few more years of life rather than to the needs of a forty-one-year-old who would go on to survive while incapacitated for more than two decades. The imminent threat of their total loss was always with them. Yet no matter how dire their economic condition may have been from time to time, Marsha always managed to save a bit from whatever funds they had at their disposal. She learned that this was a knack that she had never recognized but evidently had been born with. "I can live on spit," she once defiantly confided to me. At the same time, when she would occasionally visit her doctor for a checkup, sitting in the waiting room she might burst out in a seemingly endless stream of tears of grief and desperation.

Physically, of course, Marsha could not do it all on her own. She and Greg engaged Celia, a young black woman from the Caribbean without any special nursing credentials but who became as vitally needed and devoted to Greg as any one of his own family could be. (This was not the first time I had observed such wonderful qualities in someone from the Third World whose culture in this respect was infinitely superior to our own.) To the credit of both women, not one bed sore developed in their charge over the twenty-five years of their care to this totally bedridden man.

Like other components of a meaningful life in society, Greg's friends and colleagues gradually deserted him. There was one physician in particular, a very religious individual with clergyman credentials, who lived only a few minutes away from Greg's home. They had been very close during their years of training and had often socialized thereafter. Never once did he visit Greg throughout this time. Oddly enough, even among doctors who deal every day with disease and death there are some who feel so threatened by it when it strikes so close to home that they respond in this manner.

For my own part, having been one of Greg's mentors during part of his training, I felt a special obligation. Even so, I fell short in my own estimation. Three or four visits a year did not compensate for the growing isolation surrounding Greg. On the few occasions when I did break away from my own very busy professional and private life, I learned never to ask Greg how he was doing. I always knew that the answer would invariably be, "Worse."

Money problems, of which they rarely talked at least to me during Greg's illness, continued to plague the couple. Their parents helped out from time to time. Such concerns were also alleviated a bit for a number of years during which Greg was kept on as one of his former hospital's ECG readers. One morning a week Marsha would visit the heart station at the hospital, being sure to cajole herself into the good graces of those who worked there. She would pick up a batch of tracings for Greg to read and have them returned that afternoon. Greg's interpretations, recorded on tape, remained lucid and accurate to the very end. The few dollars of income this produced was important to them. For each reading, Celia would hold the tracing up before Greg, who would dictate his interpretation into the tape recorder. However, there came a time, some months before his death, when his voice became too weak to be heard well and the pauses on the voice-activated tape became too long because of his respiratory difficulties. He also became incapable of even holding up the microphone for this task. He was removed from the roster.

It took more than twenty-five years for Greg finally to die from his strokes and their aftermath. One day in 2003 Celia, who had developed a sixth sense about Greg, told Marsha that she believed the end was near. She did not go home that night, but huddled on a couch in the sick room to be close to her patient. We were not sure of the precise terminal event that triggered his demise, but less than twenty-four hours later Greg stopped breathing.

What, I always wondered, was the real nature of Gregg's illness once the aneurysm had been clipped and further bleeding prevented? Clinically it seemed like a slow-motion version of Lou Gehrig's disease (amyotrophic lateral sclerosis): the prolonged loss of motor function despite the preservation of mental acuity, making the patient all too aware of his plight. To me Greg's illness seemed even worse. AML patients usually succumb within a few years, while Greg's decline exceeded two decades. Was it an auto-immune disease? Had his immunological system come to identify his own neurons as the enemy and attack them forthwith? Was it a chronic inflammatory process of an unidentified nature that was the culprit?

I never received a satisfactory explanation. What I did learn from this experience was something about the tenacity to endure in a patient who had suffered so many bodily assaults. I learned that such a tragedy does not involve the patient alone. I learned that all those near and dear to such a patient suffer along with him, each in his own way. And I learned of the incredible depths of strength and devotion that this particular tragedy revealed in the woman who had chosen to be with her husband until death did them part.

21

A LETTER

A DIFFERENT KIND OF MEDICINE

It had been more than sixty years since I had last seen or spoken with Sunny (Sonja), but she had never completely faded from my memory. She was recalled to me via Helen, a friend of my kid brother Cliff, now in his mid-sixties. Cliff was introduced to Sunny when both were guests at Helen's home, and they began to compare their backgrounds. Both, it turns out, had been raised in Manhattan's Washington Heights, not far from the New York end of the George Washington Bridge. Sunny, however, was much closer in age to me than to Cliff and, it turns out, our paths had crossed in the past. When I learned of this connection, I looked forward to reminiscing with her about it. My other brother, Chick, two years my senior, had not been included within this circle of friends, and Cliff, seven years younger than I, was barely out of kindergarten at the time of my encounters with this long-lost acquaintance.

Sunny, it appears, had taken the social fast track following the early years in Washington Heights, entering what was then called café society, a far cry from the more pedestrian pursuits of her former "playmates." While mingling with the socially elite, she had seen several husbands come and go and met a lot of glamorous people, one of whom was the mutual friend, Helen. Now Sunny, like me well into her seventies, was living in Florida, with occasional trips to the Big Apple for cultural sustenance. What I was called upon to supply at the time the link was reestablished was not a lot of reminiscences but some badly needed professional advice about a choice of oncologic surgeons in Florida for the cancer that had recently been discovered in Sunny. I gladly assisted her in this, providing the names of several excellent candidates. For the time being nostalgia had to take a back seat to more pressing problems of a life-threatening nature.

A year passed, and I then learned that following surgery Sunny's tumor had metastasized and she was now undergoing chemotherapy. Things did not look good. I wondered if there was anything further I could do. There was certainly nothing more I could contribute as a physician, but it occurred to me that a letter from me might be helpful in cheering her up. On the other hand, I worried that such a communication might only drive her deeper into the natural depression that one so desperately ill must have been experiencing. I asked Helen about it and she encouraged me to write. And so I did.

Dear Sunny,

I persist in calling you this because it was always as Sunny, not Sonja, that I have remembered you as the teenage vamp of Fort Washington Avenue.

It was definitely December 6th, my birthday, but I am having trouble getting the exact year right. As for 1939, that would put me back to the age of 10, too early a time for my pubescent fantasies to take hold. By the time I was entering college in 1946 I had outgrown them although not forgotten them. So the day etched in my memory falls somewhere between 1940 and 1944 as best as I can estimate.

I was awakened that morning fully cognizant of my having gained a year even though none of my family seemed to remember. Throughout the day I steamed inwardly at their criminal neglect of this anniversary. The one compensation of the day was meeting that afternoon at a Fort Washington apartment in the 170s with a bunch of kids to play games. Was it your place? In any case for me the pièce de resistance was you, for whom I had been lusting from afar for some time—as well as a kid that age *can* lust. At the time you wore your hair in bangs, as I recall, beneath which your flashing eyes and devilish smile were irresistible.

We were playing Spin the Bottle or Post Office, the rules of both I can no longer recall. The point is that my turn had finally come to plant my longing lips upon yours. At the very moment I was about to leave the main conclave and enter another room where you awaited my passionate embrace, my older brother Chick appeared and told me that I was already late for dinner and had to come home at once. So I never "had my way with you." On the way home I berated my brother for forgetting my birthday and, as we entered the apartment at 617 West 170th Street I was already blurting out my indignation as the door began to open. I was greeted by a loud Happy Birthday cheer. It was a surprise party they had been planning all along.

I think this was the last time that I saw you, Sunny, but it is one of the most intense memories of my youth that I retain. Men really are more romantic than women, I believe. I suppose you learned of the Weisse connection from Cliff, who was only a small child at the time. I gather you met him through Helen.

What has happened in the last sixty years? Chick died accidentally at the age of thirty. Cliff has enjoyed a successful career in the theatre. I went to New York University in the Bronx as a pre-med but did not enter medical school (Downstate in Brooklyn) until my third try after almost five years during which I attempted to work in television and spent two years in the Air Force during the Korean War (1952–1954). I have had a great run in medicine, winding up as a Professor of Medicine at the New Jersey Medical School at the time of my retirement from full-time status in 1997. I still go in to the hospital once a week to read echocardiograms (ultrasound studies of the heart) and to keep abreast of current developments I still subscribe to seven of the fourteen journals that previously were delivered to my door each month. I have had some success as a medical historian and have six books to my credit. I am working on some more.

My private life was interrupted by testicular cancer as a third year medical student. I was very lucky and have survived this. However, I did marry later than I might have otherwise, finding a wonderful Dutch-American girl, Laura van Raalte, among my medical students. It would be called harassment now but it was romance then. We have been married thirty-seven years and have had two great kids. One is an English teacher in Sudbury, Mass., who was married last June and is expecting our first grandchild next May. Our son, Chick (after his deceased uncle), is a veterinary surgeon on the faculty of the University of Pennsylvania and engaged in some very interesting research. I would like to see him "hitched" as well, given the current security of his position and the clear path ahead. Laura is a practicing radiologist, very bright and hard working. Twelve years younger than I, she will probably continue working for a few years more as long as she continues to enjoy it.

I was hoping to meet with you and compare notes as well as follow up on friends we may have had in common. I don't believe our circle of friends was the same back then, each of us lying at the periphery of the other's contacts of the time, but it would be worth a try. I would be very interested in learning of your own adventures in life. As a friend of Helen, you must have had many of them.

Helen told me of your lousy luck with the cancer and I am sure that the treatment you are undergoing puts you under the weather for most of the time. Therefore, do not feel compelled to reply right away—or ever, if you so choose. I just wanted you to know that someone who "knew you when" never forgot you and is now rooting in your corner for your recovery.

All the best,
Allen

For several weeks there was no response to this letter, and I wondered if I had done the right thing. Then one day this appeared in the mail:

My dear friend,
The contents of your letter brought me much needed healing. I continue to read it. It's my medicine—as I continue to heal.

Thank you, Allen.
Sunny

"To cure sometimes, to relieve often, to comfort always."[*]

---

[*] *Guerir quelquefois, soulanger souvent, consoler toujours.* This folk saying, dated to the fifteenth century or earlier, is inscribed on Gutzon Borglum's statue of Dr. Edward Livingston Trudeau at Saranac Lake, N.Y. (M. B. Strauss, *Familiar Medical Quotations.* Boston: Little Brown, 1968, 410.)